SACRED CYCLES
THE SPIRAL OF
WOMEN'S WELL-BEING

By

Sara Wickham

Free Association Books

FA^B

Published in the United Kingdom 2004
by Free Association Books
57 Warren Street W1T 5NR

© 2004 Sara Wickham

British Library Cataloguing in Publication Data
A catalogue record for this book is available from the British Library

Produced by Bookchase (UK) Ltd
Printed by Publidisa

ISBN   1 853437 34 4

L.D.: SE-3466-2004 in Spain

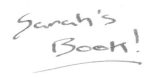
Sarah's Book!

Contents

Acknowledgements

This book has had so many midwives (both literally and metaphorically) that it seems a little unfair that there is only one name on the cover. I owe a huge thank-you to many people, including:

- All of the women who shared their experiences with me, and helped me understand a bit about what it was to experience womanhood and women's cycles from within different kinds of bodies and journeys.
- My partner, Ishvar Sheran, for his love, support, massages and ability to be eternally kind and understanding about having a woman in his life who needs space to write, insists on moon lodging, and occasionally calls him at one in the morning because one of her friends is having a crisis and we have decided that the only solution is for him to get up and drive over with more wine...
- My Mum, Rita Wickham, and all of her family and friends, for joining with me in the journey of her quilt.
- A multitude of friends who have answered my questions, read and commented on chapters and generally shared aspects of the journey of this book with me; Lorna Davies, Debbie Willett, Peggy Lee, Penny Champion, Lucyann Ashdown, Janice Marsh-Prelesnik, Janice Bass, Michel Odent, Sue Jack, Jane Evans, James Ashdown, Mary Stewart, Ruth Deery, Lynn Walcott, Tricia Anderson, Elizabeth Woolfenden and Mary Seager.
- The women, some of whom are also my friends, whose own work on similar topics has inspired some of the chapters in here: Elizabeth Davis, Robbie Davis-Floyd, Ina May Gaskin, Mirkka Lahdenperä and Carol Leonard. Special thanks to Susun Weed and Ash Tree Publishing, who have kindly allowed me to use Susun's "Six Steps of Healing", more information on which can be found at www.susunweed.com
- The Association for Improvements in the Maternity Services (AIMS), who have allowed me to adapt some of the text in "What's Right For Me? Making Decisions in Pregnancy and Birth" for Chapter 15.

- Sophie Bérubé, Yvon Malette and Les Éditions David, who have kindly given permission for the inclusion of some of Sophie's poems at the beginning of Chapters 16, 17 and 27. These poems were all originally published in *La trombe sacrée* and are copyright (2002) by Les Éditions David, Ontario.
- Trevor Brown, Free Association Books and Michel Odent for their belief in this book, and Margaret Casey at Bookchase for friendly and super-efficient editorial support.
- Finally, and by no means least, I would like to thank Green and Black's and Mister Booja Booja for making dairy-free chocolate without which my life would be a lot less rich.

A Note About Health and Responsibility

One of the major threads in this book explores the idea that women have more knowledge about what our bodies need than we generally think, and I firmly believe that we should each consider taking responsibility for our own health, perhaps in conjunction with others whose philosophy and/or expertise we value. The experiences of other women and discussion of a range of healing modalities and specific treatments are offered in that spirit; as ideas for further research and exploration rather than as specific recommendations for treatment.

Chapter 1

Women, Spirals and Patchwork Quilts

"There's beauty in the patterns of life"
(How to Make an American Quilt)

"If we are to achieve a richer culture, rich in contrasting values, we must recognize the whole gamut of human potentialities, and so weave a less arbitrary social fabric, one in which each diverse gift will find a fitting place."
(Margaret Mead)

Have you ever played the game where everybody had to decide what kind of animal or building or shape she would be? One of my friends once ran late into a meeting where we were already deciding what animal we would be. She was rushed, hot and frazzled, but still quick thinking enough to immediately answer, "I'm a headless chicken!"

Even after taking a while to ponder, I still don't know what kind of animal this book might be, but I know for sure that, if it had to be a thing, or a piece of art, it would be a patchwork quilt. Each of the chapters is a different, but complementary, piece of fabric, exploring a different aspect of women's cycles and spirals. Some of the fabrics celebrate the spirals in women's lives, and of women's power to be at the centre of their life's journey, while others highlight how women and women's cycles have been viewed by different societies over a period of time and raise questions about how we might prefer to define our own cycles. Some fabrics have been almost entirely designed by me, some include patterns crafted by other thinkers and writers, and some are rooted in the experiences of women who have never written their experiences down but who kindly shared their thoughts with me for this project.

The threads which spiral through the chapters and hold the quilt together are ideas, some of which look at some of the other aspects of life in the twenty-first century, including the ways in which we know, and the practical realities of how we might deal with problems, make decisions or bring more celebration of our cycles into our hectic modern lives.

As a quilt, this book would probably be quite varied in colour, and it would have a mixture of symmetry and chaos in the way the fabric was pieced together, both of which, as with all art, will tell you as much about the craftswoman as the piece itself. In case you'd like to know a bit more about me, I am a woman, a granddaughter, a daughter, a sister, a lover, a midwife, a teacher, a researcher, a writer and a friend. I like dairy-free chocolate, champagne and pink wine, being with my partner, mushrooms, rice and beans, travelling, spending time with my friends, making things, cooking, and celebrating the different seasons of the year (not necessarily in that order!). I am passionate about helping women to understand that they are the experts in their bodies and lives and I have written this book because I want to share some of what I have learned with other women ~ and with men who would like to get to know us better.

You won't find every kind of fabric in this book; it was never intended to be the source of everything you could ever want to know about being a woman in a woman's body. If that had been my intention, you would be holding a very fat book in your hands instead of this one. In any case, lots of other people have written really good books about all kinds of different things from a number of perspectives, and I've included some examples of other books and information you might want to look at in different areas. Also, I don't think of myself as any kind of expert on your body. Along with other so-called 'health professionals', I might know about how women's bodies work in a general way, but that doesn't mean I or anybody else have any clue as to what it means to live your life in your body.

What I have done over the past couple of years is talk to as many women as I can about what it is like to be in their bodies in this modern world, and about how their life journeys are unfolding. So this book draws upon the experiences of lots of different women, who are each on their own journeys. I invited groups of women to share their experiences with me ~ and each other ~ in women's circles. These took place in different women's homes, some during the day over coffee and cakes, and some in the evenings, around fires, sometimes with wine. I also talked to some women individually, and there were others with whom it was impractical to meet, and so we 'talked' via e-mail. This book is based on the experiences of over 100 women, ranging in age from their teens to their eighties, and from a wide variety of backgrounds. Some of these women's words are directly quoted in this book, sometimes alongside pseudonyms which the women chose themselves. In other places, I have collated the views of several women into one voice ~ yet the fabric itself is still theirs.

One of the key threads in this book explores some of the ideas that exist around how we "know" things, for instance about our bodies. We live in a society where scientific and medical research seems to be valued above all other ways of knowing, including our experiences, intuition, common-sense, or body wisdom. I teach student midwives how to understand medical and scientific research, and I think it can be a very valuable form of knowledge. However, I also think it is over-rated in modern society, which, as I said, doesn't always value other ways of knowing.

Well-conducted research can often tell us useful things about what the general trend is in large groups of people; we know, for instance, that the average menstrual cycle lasts for around 28 days. However, just because this is the average length, it does not mean that this will be the length of every woman's menstrual cycle. Similarly, midwives have tools that help us calculate when a baby is 'due' to be born, yet only three or four per cent of babies actually arrive on this day. Research is often more about mapping and predicting general trends than about giving specific, individual answers. Perhaps we need to learn to use this kind of research as a guide to the range of what is normal, rather than as fixed 'facts', which we then find don't fit with our personal situation or with what feel right to us.

The difference between 'fixed' and 'fluid' ideas has always been interesting to me. It is partly why I enjoy exploring the idea of spirals, which a number of other people have also used as an image when describing aspects of women's lives. Spirals are common in nature, unlike the straight lines of modern life, which are a human invention. The shells of many sea creatures and garden snails grow in a spiral pattern, as do sunflower seeds, pine cones and pineapples, cauliflower florets and the petals of flowers, including echinacea, the plant which is supportive of our human immune systems. Mathematicians have realised that many of the spiral patterns in nature can be described by a particular sequence of numbers, named after Fibonacci, a thirteenth century Italian mathematician. These Fibonacci numbers can be found in the growth of tree branches, planetary orbits, birds' songs, and the number of baby rabbits born over a given period of time!

Spirals can also be used as a metaphor for the different experiences women encounter during their lives. During the years that we menstruate, each month takes us through new experiences, while our body's cycle continues. Each time we bleed, we return to the same place in our menstrual cycle, while having also moved on in our lives, our relationships and our learning. So, while we call it a cycle, it might be more accurately termed the menstrual spiral, as we begin each month having grown and changed since the last.

Sometimes life can feel like a helter-skelter; you are sliding down a fast-moving spiral, feeling giddy but unable to stop yourself. At other times the same helter-skelter might feel good to us if we are feeling 'on a roll' and ecstatically happy about each new day and experience. At other times it can seem as if we are climbing an endless spiral staircase, never quite reaching the top. We could be wound up like a coiled spring, whirling like a tornado, running around in ever-decreasing circles, or drifting happily on the breeze like the smoke which swirls from the chimneys in children's drawings.

We might be on different kinds of spirals at the same time in different areas of our lives. Right now, while I am writing this paragraph, it is an Autumn Saturday lunchtime and we are waiting for some friends to arrive for the weekend. I have recently returned from a couple of trips, and have spent my working week on a medium-fast helter-skelter, trying to catch up with mail and email and bits of work that needed doing urgently. My personal life is in a happy, gently up-swirling spiral, and I spent yesterday evening with some of my best women friends and experienced some peak spiralling moments as we laughed and enjoyed each other's company. But one of my challenges at the moment is to learn how not to let my work spiral out of control, as I always have several projects to finish, and I have a tendency to suddenly find that I am on another fast helter-skelter!

Some spirals wind round gently, and it takes a while to complete the part that is almost a circle. Others are tighter; you return to the same spot more quickly, but it might take more revolutions before you reach the end. Some, like the ones on old barber's poles, create the illusion of moving eternally upwards, while actually being relatively short in themselves. And some spirals take you upwards for a while before reaching a point where they suddenly swoop down, like a roller coaster, and bring you back to the beginning again. If you are the kind of person who likes to imagine, there is probably a shape to be found for most of the patterns we experience in our life journeys.

There are some aspects of women's life journeys which I haven't examined specifically in this book. Included in this book are the experiences of women from varying cultural backgrounds (although all of whom are now living in Western, English-speaking cultures), of varying social class, sexual orientation and spiritual and religious beliefs. I talked with women who are survivors of abuse and women who have backgrounds and personal experiences which were dramatically individual. I deliberately chose not to highlight these issues in this book, except where something a woman said would not make sense unless you knew more about her. I made this decision partly because I was interested in looking at the common threads which are shared by women, who all have unique personal experiences, but also because I feel that each of these areas deserves more attention than I could give it here.

The next couple of chapters look at one of the biggest spirals; how women's experiences have changed from very ancient times and through the advent of modern society in the West, which brought very different attitudes to women from those which were held in ancient times. The following chapter then goes on to look at the 'average' experiences of women today (bearing in mind that no-body actually *is* the average!), before looking at the different cycles of women's bodies, and the spirals of their lives.

When you write a book, you need to make decisions about what will go where, and, for want of a better idea, I have begun at the beginning of life and gone through chronologically until the end, weaving in different ideas as I go. And yet the word 'chronological' means something that is logical in terms of linear time, while as women we often prefer to work in circular time. Several writers and researchers have suggested that reading something from beginning to end fits the male brain better, and that women approach things like books in different ways. There is, of course, no reason why you have to read this book in the order it is presented; you can also think of the book as a spiral, and you might like to start with the chapters that look more interesting to you, and then work forwards till you reach the end and then begin again at the beginning, or backwards from the end, or in any other way that pleases you! It often seems to me that one of the most important things we need to do as women today is to find out what most pleases us, and then do it with passion!

Chapter 2

Ancient Herstory ~ Wondering How it Was

"For an unforgettable moment, ... I felt a oneness with all mothers who had even given birth, and to mothers all over the world who were labouring and giving birth with me that night. For a fleeting moment, I saw all of us reaching deep inside for strength to break through the mental and physical limitations which we, as maidens, had assumed to exist."

(England and Horowitz 1998: 9)

With these words, Midwife Pam England describes her own experience of labour, and offers an insight into why she works so hard enabling other women to find connections, in their minds, bodies and hearts, with all of the generations of women who have successfully birthed before them. She, among many other midwives, sets out to help women become conscious of the fact that they can give birth and that their body is a marvellous creation. In these days of doctor-controlled and technology-focused childbearing, the realisation that their body has been designed to successfully give birth can be quite a revelation for some women ~ and make all the difference to their experience.

If those women who came before us had not each successfully birthed the next generation, we would, of course, not even be here today to wonder about them. It is always a marvel to me to realise that every single one of my 'great' grandmothers managed to give birth to at least one baby in her lifetime, and that we each come from a wondrously successful lineage of birthing women. With this in mind, wondering about those generations of women who lived before the dawn of our modern world might be a good place to begin.

In a society where many facets of everyday life, including the calendar, have developed alongside the male-based worldview, there is a tendency to begin histories by thinking back only a couple of thousand years, or to Biblical times. Yet humans flourished on the Earth long before this time, and we could travel back in time many thousands of years and still find recognisable ancestors. We might have to acknowledge that our interpretations of the archaeology we find from different periods are influenced by our own beliefs and worldview, but there are a few things we could probably say with some confidence.

We can be fairly certain, for instance, that ancient women (and ancient men) would have relied more on storytelling and passing on knowledge by talking to each other than we do. Today, we have massive repositories of written and stored knowledge in the form of libraries, databanks and the Internet, and you can find out how to make bread through any of these means. There are even machines which can make it for you, if you just put all of the right things inside them. Yet in ancient times your major source of knowledge would have been your mother, and the other women around you. You might have built upon their knowledge within your own experience, and passed that on to your daughters, or you could have ignored their advice and used trial-and-error to figure it out for yourself, but you certainly couldn't go to the back of your dwelling and grab a recipe book or nip online to search for a web page.

Some people view the ancient world as a hard, barbaric, and dangerous place, where life was uncomfortable, perhaps shorter than now, and people fought mercilessly over land. These people may be very happy they live in our modern world, with its technology and development. Others see ancient society through a more romantic lens, and yearn to return to times where nature was untainted by technology, with simpler values and kinship ties being the order of the day. Even where we acknowledge that technology has made our lives less arduous and more fun, legends about places such as Atlantis and the Garden of Eden fuel the idea that a simpler life led closer to nature might ultimately be more fulfilling.

Over the past couple of decades, researchers and historians have begin to look at the ancient world with a lens which takes more account of the role and experience of women than ever before. The very fact that history ("*his story*") is so named should give us a clue that this area has mainly been studied from a male perspective, and the view that women did not do much of note in the past is being overtaken by a realisation that some ancient societies were much more matrifocal, or woman-focused, than ours is today.

Riane Eisler (1988) argues that most ancient societies were based around a *partnership model*, where women and men worked in harmony, rather than the *dominator model* of modern society, where women have not attained total equality with men. She points to evidence such as the stone *Venus* statues depicting triumphantly naked women, who may be menstruating or birthing (previously interpreted by some male historians as being erotic imagery for ancient men), cave paintings showing the spiritual and ceremonial importance of women and the role of red ochre, symbolising menstrual blood, in ancient funeral rites. The discovery of ancient and powerful Mother-Goddess figures, sometimes together with their Father-God counterparts, is in stark contrast to older views of history which have suggested that women were "designed" to be subservient to men and that they have always played a lesser role in society.

The work of women like Riane Eisler suggests that, in ancient matrifocal societies, birth and motherhood were respected and revered, which creates a very different view of the beginnings of humanity from the one we might have previously taken. A society that reveres mothers is unlikely to have treated human mothers in the ways they are sometimes treated today. There have been times in my life as a midwife where I have despaired to see new mothers being left alone for long periods because their families are too busy to help them, or women who are struggling to cope with their new baby because they are being physically or mentally abused by their partners. These are situations that I just cannot imagine occurring frequently in a society whose core values include kinship and respect for women. It is also hard to imagine a woman from an ancient society which revered the Mother-Goddess' life-giving abilities happily lying on her back with her legs in the air and allowing a man to 'deliver' her child with tools or machines while she remains relatively passive. Indeed, cave paintings of ancient women giving birth show them in upright positions, surrounded by other women.

It is not just the ability of women to give birth that seems to have earned them this respect in ancient times; their knowledge and insight would also have been more valued than it is today. Our society talks about "old wives' tales" in a derogatory way; we use this phrase to refer to something which we feel is untrue (although I have more to say about that in Chapter 24!). Yet old wives' tales have taught many young women (and men) what they needed to know about the world. Thirty thousand years ago, menopausal women would not have been seen as 'past their prime'; they are more likely to have been respected and sought out for their great wisdom and experience. In a society where young people learned at the feet of older women, these older women would have been far more valued than in a society where young people learn from books and computers, and where midwife teachers who are now university lecturers regularly teach fifty or a hundred student midwives at one time, rather than on a one-to-one basis.

These new analyses of old evidence might also mean we need to re-evaluate our beliefs around the herstory of the way women's blood and the menstrual cycle was viewed. Judy Grahn (1993) was one of the women who overturned the myth that, because menstruation is largely hidden in our modern world, this has always been the case. The word "taboo" is sometimes associated with menstruation, and she shows that this word comes from a Polynesian word meaning both "sacred" and "menstruation". How different it must have been to live in a society where having periods was considered sacred.

Grahn interprets historical evidence which others seem to have ignored showing that, in some cultures, menstrual blood was once seen as a magical substance, filled with power and mystery. Where some more recent interpretations seem to suggest that menstruating women should be segregated from the rest of the society because they are dirty, she argues that there are some cultures where, while segregation may well have been the order of the day, this was a far more positive thing for women than we have come to believe. What about if women did not segregate themselves because they felt they were dirty; but instead they segregated themselves because they understood how magical they were and wanted to tap into that magic in an all-female environment? What about if they discovered that segregation allowed them to rest and recuperate from hard work for a few days each month, while also enabling them to have a really good time with their woman friends?

A few religious traditions have been accused of promoting women's "dirtyness", inferiority and subservience as if it were a natural law. Yet how can we be sure, in the light of the emerging evidence, that this was really the way it was in ancient times? Could those men who were doing the translation or explanation have misinterpreted these works, either deliberately or in error? Perhaps these interpretations reflect the beliefs and political aspirations of their day rather than the original truth in the documents? It seems silly to throw out any belief system in its entirety because it has aspects we find uncomfortable; far more interesting to me is the way in which women and men from all different beliefs and faiths are re-evaluating their lives and their devotions as time passes and our understanding grows.

Reinterpretations of ancient herstory are coming from a number of directions, and they all seem to be pointing to a similar conclusion; that the things we women have been taught to believe about ourselves and our bodies may not be the whole truth. They may be partially true, but they may also have been re-moulded somewhat to serve the purposes of those who have held power at different times in our past. We may have missed some essential truths along the way, or lost them on our journey. The herstory spiral may not look quite like we once imagined. Ancient women seem to have been more equal and respected than we have come to think and, while we might not want to give up all of our advances and creature comforts and return there wholesale, we may be able to learn and grow by looking at how our loss of this situation has impacted on our experiences of being women today.

Chapter 3

Modern Herstory and its Impact on Women

While ancient women may have been at the centre of their societies, the subsequent modernisation, industrialisation and scientification of Western society has not been entirely positive for women. A number of people have explored this area and variously placed blame (among other things) on male-based religion (Sjöö and Mor 1987; Jaggar 1988; Arms 1994), on scientific rationalism (Abercrombie 1988) and on the men who found power by claiming that their ways of knowing were preferable (Illich 1990). Each of these things has been criticised and defended by various people at length, and my intention here is not to repeat all of those ~ the criticisms and defences ~ which can be found elsewhere, but to look at a few key facts and factors which raise important questions for women today.

It is important to realise that it is precisely because Western culture became male-focused for so many years that, until recently, people have tended to assume that things were always that way, or that this was a 'natural' state of being. As the idea that women should defer to men grew, this notion began to be incorporated into language, into the writings of the day and into laws and cultural traditions. Many of these things have been transferred into the words, books, laws and conventions which we follow today; one example being that some women still promise to obey their husbands when they marry. We need to recognise that these are not natural laws; they have evolved culturally and socially in response to historical events and changes, and we can only wonder how things might have been if the circumstances had been different.

The sixteenth and seventeenth centuries heralded a time of particular terror for women, characterised as they were by the killing of thousands of innocent women:

> *"While Michaelangelo was sculpting and Shakespeare writing, witches were burning ... Renaissance men were celebrating naked female beauty in their art, while women's bodies were being tortured and burned by the hundreds of thousands all around them."*
> (Sjöö and Mor 1987, p 309)

Women with knowledge, often about herbs, midwifery and healing, represented a political, religious and economic threat to both organised religion and the state (Brook 1976). Almost certainly this was instrumental in leading women to fear speaking out, a fear that has been passed on to generations of women through gender socialisation. Women lost faith in themselves, in their bodies, in their knowledge and in each other:

> *"History has pulverised women's psychic powers and offered up femininity on a stake and labelled witch ..."*
> (Brook 1976: 28)

How different might things have been if, instead of being persecuted for their knowledge, women had been able to pass this on to their daughters and, once ways of recording knowledge over time were developed, to write it down? We would be able to look at it now, with all of the other things we have learned in the meantime and see how useful and relevant it could be to us. As we seek to reclaim our ways of knowing, we can only wonder about the knowledge that has been lost. If women had not been set against each other during those times, would we now be better at collaborating with our sisters, rather than competing with them?

If it had been primarily men who were persecuted and killed, instead of women, how different would our society be today? Would we have been in a similar but reversed situation, with men having had to fight for the right to vote, and taking themselves off to university to read "Men's Studies"? Would modern women have no interest in books like this one, while instead men wrote about reclaiming their cycles from their own perspective, rather than women's? Would we women, as a gender, have shared power with men, or held it more carefully, or would men have been just as subjugated as women?

The loss of women's knowledge through the witch-hunts was followed by the 'age of enlightenment' of the eighteenth century, which involved massive social, political and economic changes (Giddens 1987). Modernity led to increased secularisation and scientific rationalism (Mitchell 1986) and rationalism in turn led to the view that science is the best way to gather knowledge ~ yet the initial barring of women from science meant that a whole half of humanity had no influence on this new way of thinking.

While the roots of logic and reasoning go back at least as far as the ancient Greek philosophers, it is men like Rene Descartes and Francis Bacon who are generally credited with the initial development of modern scientific thinking. In his scientific work, Bacon announced he was launching, "an aggressive male attack on women's secrets" (Sjöö and Mor 1987: 323). Helped along by Descartes' claim that there was a clear separation between the physical body and the mind (and other aspects such as the soul or spirit), the thinkers and scientists of the day began to make claims about women's bodies, which were, in turn, adopted by doctors. As recently as the nineteenth century, many doctors believed that, if women's brains were more fully developed, their ovaries would suffer (Schiebinger 1987).

The widespread idea that the male body was "the norm" and that differences in the female body are then compared to this led to the view that women's sexual organs were lesser versions of the male prototypes. As just one example, this, in turn, led to the underplaying of the size and role of the clitoris. I don't know how ancient women viewed the clitoris, but modern society's view of this amazing creation has suffered from quite incredible levels of distortion. As Sjöö and Mor (1987; 4–5) point out, "women are used to hearing the clitoris described as an 'undeveloped penis'; men are not used to thinking of the penis as an overdeveloped clitoris". Most books have described the clitoris as being an organ only a couple of centimetres in length which exists only outside a woman's body. Yet the clitoris is actually an organ with multiple aspects, including two sections which extend backwards, inside the woman's body, and bulbs which nestle alongside the vaginal opening. The clitoris also surrounds the bladder, which may explain why some of the women I talked to mentioned that they often felt sexually aroused when they really needed to pee.

When Helen O'Connell, an Australian urologist, published the work she and her colleagues had carried out on the clitoris (1998), there was a fair amount of media interest. They weren't the first to point out that our view of the clitoris was distorted; anatomists had known about these structures for years, yet somehow this knowledge hadn't made it into textbooks and education systems. Her concern was that, although the microscopic structures of the penis were well understood, those of the clitoris had never been studied. If we remained ignorant of these structures, she argued, surgeons could not take care to preserve them when they were carrying out surgical operations in this area, such as hysterectomy.

In some ways it is not surprising that the (mainly internal) structure of the clitoris wasn't understood until people began looking inside other people's bodies. Yet even when Renaissance men (who excluded women from their universities) began to dissect human bodies, they based their studies of women on the assumption that women's genitals were based on men's genitals, but turned inside-out. They weren't looking for structures which were unique to women. To be fair, we should remember that we are all products of the belief systems in which we grew up, and that, because they used the bodies of criminals for their dissections, they had far more male than female bodies to study. Unfortunately, by the time anatomy became more scientific, Victorian values held that women's sexual organs were not suitable topics for research, and Freudian views of female sexuality effectively put the lid on this debate for several decades (Bennett 1993). As a result, it is only very recently that we are becoming aware of how biased our understanding of female sexuality in general and the clitoris in particular has been.

While modern times and scientific thinking brought great improvements to some aspects of people's lives, many of the advances of modernity are double-edged swords, and the development of technology is one example of this. Having a mobile phone and a car makes it much easier for me to be a midwife than in the time when my grandmother had her babies; my grandfather had to run to fetch the midwife when she was giving birth, and the midwife had to cycle to women's homes in all weather. On the other hand, there is plenty of modern technology which we may be better off without, or which is useful on occasion, but may also be used inappropriately.

The involvement of men in birth (beginning around the time of the witch-hunts) gives a good example of this. Our history books record that it was men who invented forceps, although I feel confident that female midwives then, as today, had their own ways of helping babies out when things became difficult. The development of technological ways to intervene in birth was, for the few women who genuinely need help, a good thing. For many others, however, the subsequent (and sometimes unnecessary) involvement of technology in the birth process has led to women feeling that it is doctors, rather than themselves, who are in control.

These examples show that, during the last few centuries, power has been firmly held in the hands of men, as doctors, church leaders and members of other specific professional groups ~ the vast majority of whom were male. While the impact of this situation on women is clear, the situation is changing, in more ways than one. For a start, the most powerful organisations today include multi-national companies who do not have a geographical base that can be threatened. The major stakeholders in the health care 'business' include the multi-national pharmaceutical, technology and formula milk companies. The influence of these companies on our lives can be clearly seen in the choices made by women (and men) in response to advertising, trends and spin.

However, these companies stand to lose an immense amount of money if the numbers of people seeking alternatives to Western medicine and drugs continues to grow, and if women continue to realise just how much power they hold as consumers. While Arms (1994: 60) notes that, "it is a small step from having no economic or political power to feeling and behaving like a victim", more and more women are realising that they do not have to be victims of the system and that they do hold the key to their own power.

Since the mid-nineteenth century, there have been Social Reform Movements whose concerns centred on child labour, maternity care and mothers' rights (Arms 1994). These movements continue to work today, in varied forms, to help women reclaim their bodies, cycles, health, ways of knowing and power over birth. However strongly the medical profession or other groups may influence society in terms of power, there is one type of power they will never hold ~ the power of women to give birth and nurture their children.

There exists a wider range of ideas and theories about health and well being than many women may realise. Alongside the tradition of Western medicine there exists not only 'alternative', 'traditional' or 'complementary' medicine but also a set of beliefs and practices which has come to be called the "wise woman" tradition (Weed 1989). Where Western medicine sets out to treat the symptoms of a disease, and alternative medicine often encourages people to 'clean up their act' and live healthier lives, the wise woman tradition focuses more on seeing that we are already whole and loving who we are. Where Western medicine places power in drugs and surgery and alternative traditions in the healer, wise women know that they hold their own power (Weed 1989). They might still use practices and techniques from the Western and alternative traditions, but they place themselves at the centre of their experiences; as Susun Weed points out, being a wise woman is a way of thinking, not a way of acting.

As I noted at the beginning of this chapter, many people have documented the events of modern times and the ways in which they have impacted upon women. It seems to me that we now need to take this knowledge and take a look at how this has impacted on women today (which is the subject of the next chapter) but also choose where we go with it. We need to ask ourselves some fundamental questions about our situation, about our health and cycles and about the way in which we (and others) view our bodies. We need to decide whether, for us as individuals, we believe in pharmaceutical drugs, natural remedies, technology, healthy living, creating our own reality, surgical intervention ~ or all of the above. We need to decide whether we are happy with the consequences of modernity ~ and, if not, what kind of a world we want to live in. We need to consider whether we are content with the status quo, or whether more of us are wise women than we might have thought.

Chapter 4

Twenty-First Century Girl

This is a story of four women who all live in the Western world today. Their names are Violet, Joan, Laura and Skye, and each of these women gave birth to the next. Violet was born in the early part of the twentieth century, and Skye was born at the beginning of the twenty-first. There is, of course, no such person as the 'average' girl or woman; we are all on unique journeys shaped and coloured by our individual experiences. Yet there may be some general things we can say about the experience of being a woman in Western culture today which will apply to the experience of many women, albeit in different ways. The stories of Violet, Joan, Laura and Skye are an amalgam of the stories of a number of different women from these four generations.

Violet was born in rural England in 1920. She grew up working hard, looking after her brothers and sisters and helping her own mother around the house. Her mother was often too busy looking after the youngest child to pay much attention to the older children, and Violet knew that the best thing she could do was to be "seen and not heard" as much as possible. She learned quickly that the needs of others were more important than her own and, with a clear understanding that women were inferior to men, promised to honour and obey her husband when she got married to a local boy at the age of sixteen.

Violet's mother had told her nothing about the workings of her body; she came home bleeding and worried one day, thinking she had a dreadful illness. She recalls her mother seemed somewhat annoyed that Violet wanted to discuss this when she was obviously busy with the new baby. Worried, Violet confided in one of her friends, who was able to share a little more information with her. Her friend had learned that once a month a "curse" would hit her body, causing her to bleed, and that it was linked to the fact that she would one day have babies, although she was not entirely sure how this would happen. They both understood that this "curse" was something slightly shameful, to be hidden away from everybody, and barely talked even to each other about it after that.

Violet did not, however, see her menstrual cycle as being within the remit of the medical profession until much later in her life. As a child, she had been taught to have great respect for doctors and nurses, among other professional groups. She believed that they understood far more about what was going on inside her body than she did. Violet's respect for health care professionals remains so great that, to this day, if a doctor disagreed with her about where she was feeling a pain, she would wonder if her own senses were wrong.

When Violet became pregnant with her first child, she was not entirely sure how the baby would come out, although she knew it had something to do with her bottom. She also had no idea when the baby would come out. She did not want to bother the midwife with such silly questions, so again asked around her friends what they thought. Sadly, most of her friends knew no more than she did, and none had yet had babies of their own.

Violet gave birth to Joan in her bedroom at home, lying on her left side, with the local midwife in attendance and blackout curtains up the windows. Her labour was fairly fast, and the birth was easy. The idea of using pain relief for labour was unknown in the village where Violet lived, and even where it was available Violet thinks that to use it would have been a failing. She bit the pillow when the pains were really bad. She spent the next couple of weeks lying-in in her bedroom and a few of the local women came in to help with the baby and cook for her husband. It would never have occurred to Violet not to breastfeed Joan, or the other babies that came after her; apart from anything else, artificial milk would have been an expensive extravagance which they could ill-afford. It also never occurred to Violet that she might not be able to breastfeed, she got on with this as she got on with everything else in her life, and Joan grew into a happy and healthy baby.

Joan remembers her own childhood being quite strict, and learning that her place was primarily in the home, although later she was also expected to contribute to the family income. Her only memory now of learning about her menstrual cycle was when she complained of a series of headaches and Violet thrust a medical leaflet at her. Joan's friend Pam had an older sister who had always tended to take more care of their needs than their mothers, and Pam's sister explained what she knew, which Joan now realises was not really that much either! Joan gave up studying biology at school when she was about thirteen, and had always assumed she would have learned more there, until she learned from a friend recently that the biology teacher had only taught rabbit reproduction! Where Violet didn't seem to feel that she deserved information, and was quite stoic about her experiences, Joan realised ~ now and then ~ that there was information to be had, but was often frustrated in her efforts to get it. She learned a bit from talking with her friends, as she had with Pam's sister, although she came to realise that, while the intentions were always good, not everything she learned that way was entirely accurate.

When she was sixteen, Joan went out to work, to help support the family, and spent a couple of years having fun as a single woman before she met and married her husband. He came from the nearby town where Joan worked. They married, and she went on the pill for a few years so they could both work and save up money to buy a house before they started a family. The pill was very new and many women remember being quite excited about taking it:

> *"I thought it was great ... it was quite exciting really ... here was this thing that would let me get pregnant only when I wanted to ... I thought those scientists were just brilliant. My friend, though, her doctor wouldn't let her go on the pill, she was married too but he [the doctor] was a bit old-fashioned."*
>
> (Jeannie)

At around the same time, Violet began to experience hot flashes and heavy bleeding, which she knew were something to do with "the change of life". Again, she saw this as something to cope with, not wanting to bother anybody else. Joan had a different opinion, but it wasn't until Violet nearly passed out that she finally agreed to go and see the doctor, who diagnosed a fibroid. She immediately agreed to the treatment recommended by the doctor, and was one of the most well-behaved patients he had ever met. She did not question him once, even when he brought nine or ten medical students to her room and asked if they could all examine her. Although Violet did not enjoy this at all, she felt that it would be the right thing to do and that he wouldn't have asked her if it wasn't really important. Violet went on pick up an infection, which the nurses told Joan may have been from all the examinations, yet Violet did not believe this and blamed herself for not taking good enough care of herself beforehand.

Joan felt too unwell to visit Violet in hospital very much towards the end of her stay because she was again pregnant, having experienced a miscarriage about a year before. She was relieved to be experiencing morning sickness because she hadn't with her first pregnancy, and her family doctor told her that feeling nauseous was a good sign that the baby was OK. As Violet had before her, Joan felt that the doctors knew more about her body than she did, although she had begun to realise from her friend's experience of trying to go on the pill that different doctors had different approaches and that there was a range of different medical opinions.

Joan went to antenatal classes with a group of other local women, and learned a fair bit about the biology of how babies came out, but very little about what to do with them once they had:

> *"There was just a complete shortage of information about that;*
> *they told you all about the birth and what they were going to*
> *do to you, but nothing much else."*
>
> (Carol)

Laura was born in a small maternity home, with Joan lying on her back, the midwife in attendance and her husband watching TV with the doctor in the waiting room. Joan used gas and air for the pain, and the midwife cut her to allow the baby's head out, which Joan knew was routine (for they had told her it would happen in the antenatal classes) but is still traumatised about today. Laura was taken away to the nursery, and was only brought back to Joan when she needed feeding. Joan left the maternity home feeling ill-equipped to deal with this tiny baby, yet also feeling she had got off fairly lightly as one of her friends had given birth at around the same time after being induced in the hospital as her baby was overdue. Her friend had been left alone with agonising pains from the drugs she had been given and the staff did not believe her when she said she wanted to push; the midwife only came back into the room as the baby's head was almost out.

Laura spent a fair amount of time at the doctor's surgery when she was a child; she had countless courses of antibiotics for various ear and throat infections, and quite liked the attention of it all. Joan did not believe that her knowledge of Laura's health and well-being was adequate and often needed the reassurance of a 'professional'. Laura's biology teacher was less interested in rabbit reproduction than Joan's friend's teacher had been and covered human reproduction in depth, as did the school nurse. Any gaps in Laura's knowledge were filled by the problem pages in the old copies of women's magazines which Violet used to hoard in an old magazine rack for Laura and her cousins to read when they went to stay. Laura well remembers the TV advertisements portraying periods as something to be hidden away, and strangely used blue water to demonstrate the absorbency of different kinds of tampons. Joan did attempt to talk to Laura about some of the things Violet had not told her, but realised that Laura seemed to know more than she did, and felt inadequate.

Laura learned a lot about menstrual cycles, birth and menopause from these different sources, although she now realises that much of it was focused on these things being "medical":

> *"It wasn't like, this is normal, this is what happens and it's OK ...*
> *it was often all about what can go wrong, what is abnormal, not*
> *what's normal and here it is and this is a part of being a woman.*
> *If someone from another planet read it, they would probably*
> *think it was a bad idea to be a women on earth ... it was a bit*
> *abnormal."*
>
> (Lauren)

Laura's school nurse separated girls and boys for talks about this kind of thing, and Laura learned that contraception was her responsibility as a woman, and that she would be well advised to accept this responsibility rather than leave it to a boyfriend or partner who would not have to deal with the impact and consequences of an unwanted pregnancy. Possibly, she feels, as a result of this, Laura went on the pill at the age of seventeen, although she did not have a boyfriend at the time. But she was planning to go to university, and wanted to be prepared.

Joan started to go through her menopause while Laura was at university, and went straight to the doctor for help. At first, the doctor said that this was a natural thing and she should just get on with it, but Joan was not happy with this, so a few months later made an appointment with another doctor and got hormone replacement therapy. She took this for three years until she became concerned about the reports of side effects in the papers and on television, when she decided to stop.

Laura married Peter a couple of years after they graduated, and they, like Laura's parents before them, made sure their careers were well established before they decided to start a family. Skye was conceived a few years later on a beach in St Tropez, when her parents made love towards the end of their holiday there. When she got back home, Laura went to see her family doctor, and had a positive pregnancy test. Laura had an early ultrasound scan on the advice of her doctor, which Skye did not like very much, but which Laura thought was a good idea because she would then know exactly when the baby was due.

When Laura then went to see the midwife, she asked if Laura had thought about having her baby at home or in the local birth centre, and when Laura said she hadn't, the midwife wrote down that she was having the baby in the hospital. Laura thought nothing more of this. She went to classes at the hospital with her husband during pregnancy, where they met some nice people, but didn't learn a lot that they hadn't already read in books. She remarked to Peter once or twice that it almost seemed as if the midwives who were running the classes were trying to teach the women how to be "good girls" during their labour and birth.

Laura had two more scans during her pregnancy, one of which slightly worried her because the technician couldn't see part of the baby and therefore couldn't tell her that everything was definitely OK. Violet privately thought that all of this ultrasound and technology might be going a bit over the top; in her day, women learned to cope with problems and they accepted that babies occasionally had problems. But she would never dream of arguing with something a doctor might suggest. She had recently been in hospital again, to have surgery on her hip, which she broke after she slipped on ice in the winter. She was, again, a "star patient", recovering more quickly than anyone had thought possible and, at the age of 80, keen to get home to visit the 'elderly' lady up the road.

Laura's baby, Skye, was born in hospital. The birth seemed to go well, and Skye was healthy, but, towards the end, Laura didn't really feel she had a lot to do with it. Her labour was quite long, although Skye wasn't distressed, and in the end the doctor came in and said he was going to "lift out" baby Skye with forceps. It felt to Laura as if her insides were being pulled out. She went home after two days, as the ward was busy, and tried to breastfeed but never really figured it out. She felt the midwives' visits after the baby was born were a bit pointless; all they did was upset Skye by taking her clothes off each time to check in her nappy and, as the midwives always talked about how many visits they had to do that day, Laura never really felt there was time to ask questions. When one midwife suggested it might be an idea to give Skye a bottle so Laura could get some rest, she felt too tired to ask whether it was true that this could interfere with breastfeeding. The next time Laura tried, Skye wouldn't breastfeed at all so Laura gave up and asked Peter to go out to stock up on bottles and formula.

Laura thinks she might ask for a bit more information about the birth centre when she gets pregnant again, as she has heard that you can stay there for a bit longer afterwards and she likes the idea of this. She feels she might like to try to breastfeed again next time, but isn't really sure whether she can. Laura sometimes wonders if it might have been easier for Violet's generation, where the choices were more limited, as she spends so much time trying to decide what is right for Skye that she feels she has little time for herself. She doesn't believe that it is right to simply do what professionals suggest, but knows that, when things go wrong, there is little else you can do except let them take over. Violet wishes she would have talked more to Laura, or that she could have been around when Laura was trying to breastfeed, but she didn't like to interfere, or to disagree with what the midwife said.

Skye is learning what it is to be born female in the twenty-first century, and will, as her mother and grandmothers before her, be shaped by their ideas, the social norms and the attitudes of the world around her. Who can know what her choices will be, or how her life will evolve ...

* * * * * * *

Who is Ms average?

The characters in this story were based on an amalgamation of women's stories, yet none of these women are average in themselves. The following accounts are based on the experiences of a group of real women in their late twenties who had been friends since their schooldays.

While not representing all of the possible experiences and social situations of women today, they do highlight some of the main issues that came up for the women I talked to for this book. In the context of this story, these women could be considered to be Laura's friends...

Fran married the boy next door, and they have had three children. She has always liked the idea of going back to study, but has not yet managed to persuade her husband that this would be a good idea. He has a good job and feels that she needs to be there for the children. Fran feels satisfied with her life, if a bit unfulfilled on a personal level.

Carlie's partner is West Indian and his grandmother is a traditional midwife. When they spent a month there a few years ago, Carlie (who had originally worked in a travel agency) fell in love with the old lady and became passionate about the idea of being a midwife herself. She is currently undertaking a three-year midwifery degree, and loves the idea of being an "earth mother" one day. She hates having to work in the hospital, as she now feels that home is the safest and best place to give birth for most women. She is hoping to work as a community midwife when she qualifies, and spends a lot of time researching alternatives to Western medicine through her course and on the Internet. Carlie is on a bit of a crusade to tell other women about home birth and brings it up in conversation whenever she can; she has spent a lot of time talking Laura through her birth experience and helping her see that it might not have been her "fault" that she didn't manage to breastfeed.

Christine married straight out of school and had one baby in the local hospital a couple of years after she married. She had such a miserable time and was depressed for so long afterwards that she has vowed never to have another. She goes to her doctor every few months for a contraceptive injection and dotes on her daughter, Lizzie.

Vanessa realised at the age of sixteen that she was more interested in women than men, and has recently been attending workshops with her partner, Julie, in the hope that they can have a baby of their own. She has always been very interested in the politics of reproduction, and volunteers on a helpline for women who have had unpleasant experiences giving birth in hospital. She and Julie are torn between what they term the "natural route" and the "medical route". In many ways, they would prefer to do it themselves, but are a bit concerned about the potential for sexually transmitted infection. Yet they are fearful of the potential side effects of medical treatment and don't like the idea of giving up control of conception and birth to doctors.

Alison tries to be as supportive to Vanessa as she can, but has confessed to Vanessa that she can't really understand what the fuss is about. She had two babies in hospital, both with an epidural and would recommend it to anybody. Both times the midwife made the epidural wear off so that Alison could push the babies out herself and Alison couldn't praise the doctors and midwives highly enough. She jokingly tells both Vanessa and Carlie that they are making mountains out of molehills with all of this "natural stuff" and, having not been to university herself, wonders if all of this education is what causes the problem...

Sarah has started her own business and is living with Paul, who has three children of his own from a previous marriage. She is very happy being their weekend stepmother and not having babies of her own. She has always thought it was a very messy business and not something she wanted to experience personally. Sarah has a drawer full of drugs for PMT, which she suffers from a lot. Carlie gave her a pack of herbal tea and wheat pillow for her birthday, but she hasn't tried them yet. Sarah is already looking forward to the menopause, and plans to get some hormone replacement therapy as soon as she can. She is waiting for Paul to get a date for a vasectomy.

Amanda had an abortion while at University and has never really enjoyed sex since. She is now studying for a higher degree and trying to avoid commitment, planning instead to fill her life with a successful career in education. She is aware that some of these issues might be worth looking at, but prefers not to think about it.

* * * * * *

Clearly, Ms Average is a figment of the imagination; while the fabric of Laura, Violet and Joan was made from the threads which came up most often in women's stories, these are only some of the many threads running through women's lives. No two women have the same stories; we each have a variety of threads which are woven together in different ways, and Ms Average exists only on paper and in the minds of marketing executives...

Chapter 5

Being Born a Woman

In the first six months of her life, Skye was exposed to a variety of technology and seven different chemical substances in the name of nourishment and improving her health. She had barely recovered from being pulled from her mother's body with forceps when the cord linking her to her mother's body was cut and she was placed on a table to be "checked" and injected with vitamin K, to help her blood clot. She was glad to snuggle up with her mother and find her breast. Two days later, she was given formula milk. On the seventh day, a lancet was stuck into her foot so blood could be taken to check for disease and she was given another drug a few days later because the midwife saw she had thrush. Over the next few months she was injected with two different vaccine mixtures to protect her immune system, given infant paracetamol when she was fractious and prescribed antibiotics when she had a cold. Skye was grateful that her mother went to the trouble of buying the more expensive additive-free baby lotion.

I think it is important to say at the outset that the paragraph above is not intended to be a judgement about anybody who chooses to bottle feed, vaccinate or give drugs to their baby. All of these things have their place and goodness knows that mothers already have enough people trying to make them feel guilty; that is not my intention at all. It is, however, something of a judgement about how focused our society tends to be on using chemicals and technology to solve problems, and how poor we often are as health professionals about informing women of the different options, pros and cons of applying these drugs and machines to their new babies. How might our babies feel about this if they could better communicate with us?

As a new baby, what might it feel like to be injected with artificial sub-stances within hours of your birth, or to have a lancet or needle pushed into your tiny body to collect blood for analysis? Yet, as a new mother or father, how can you help but follow the advice of those who are 'experts' in our babies, as you struggle to make sense of the conflicting opinions swirling around us? What would our babies choose if they could? Where we used to believe that unborn and newly born babies could not learn, feel pain or interact intelligently with their environment, lots of studies have shown that this is untrue; that babies can react to individual voices, play games and form relationships even at this early stage (Chamberlain 2003). But can they tell us what their choices would be about this kind of thing?

I do often wonder what babies are thinking in those first few moments and days. I challenge anybody who has been around birth for a while not to wonder if babies sometimes seem to know much more than they can tell us. When I look into the eyes of a newborn baby, I can really relate to the idea of reincarnation; I sometimes imagine they are thinking, "Oh no, not again!" A number of other mothers and midwives agree with me that, when you see enough new people being born, you stop thinking of babies as helpless beings and start to think of them as wise spirits in tiny bodies:

> *"I will never forget that slippery, wet body being laid across mine as we met each other after labouring together for a time-less day. Instantly, her brilliant and precious eyes reminded me that she was an ancient soul in a brand-new body and her innate nature was just as evolved as mine, if not more so."*
> (Luminaire-Rosen 2000: 1)

So how can we best help these wise spirits into the earthly world? Perhaps by thinking about how we would like to be welcomed...

If you were about to take a long trip to another world, entirely new and different, how would you like to be greeted when you got there? You will, by the way, travel in a very small spaceship without much room to move and be helpless when you get to that world, having to adapt and grow used to the atmosphere and environment around you. Although you will be the expert in how to travel in your spaceship and how to exit it when you arrive, and your spaceship is 'intelligent' and will help you through this process, once you do exit you will be unable to move well in the new world and will initially rely on others for all of your needs.

When you get close to the new world, would you mind if the people there used their technology to look inside your spaceship and monitor your well-being? The technology might be noisy and might, like our ultrasound does, make you want to try to wriggle or jump away from the probe. Assuming you know you are not in danger by remaining inside for a while longer, would you rather decide when you felt ready to leave the spaceship yourself, or would you mind if your new companions decided when to get you out? What about if they felt you were taking longer to emerge than most visitors, while you might have decided you would like to rest for a while and stop your exit/entry process to take a breath ~ would you mind if they put machinery on your head and pulled you out, or if they cut the side of your spaceship wide open and pulled you quickly out of your familiar cocoon into their strange new world?

Your spaceship has been dark and the outside noise muffled. Would you rather emerge to be greeted by welcoming whispers, dim lights and gentle, soft, cradling hands, or pulled out quickly and placed on a cold surface under bright lights in a noisy room? You have a 'breathing and feeding' tube which has kept you alive for the past few months' journey, and you will need to release this at some point and learn to take nourishment in a new form. Would you rather decide when you are ready to close down this tube yourself and begin to breathe the atmosphere in the new world, or are you happy for your new companions to cut it as soon as your body has emerged?

Of course, in the real-life parallel to this, our new wise human spirits are not emerging from an inert spaceship, but from a living, breathing, feeling woman, who is connected with her 'passenger' on a deep level and who also has choices to make. In modern society, this woman may be berated for wanting to choose a more gentle birth for both her baby's sake and her own; she will often be told that she is placing her desire for a "nice experience" above her baby's well-being. I do wonder, though, if we gave more thought to what it is like to be born, and the way in which we would like to experience our birth if we were to be born again, whether more people might have more sympathy for the idea of gentle birth from the perspective of the baby.

* * * * * * *

When Skye was three, she was playing round Joan's house with three of her male cousins. Their ages ranged from two to five, and the older boys happily ran around the garden with her for a while. Laura's younger brother Andy then came outside and the boys immediately wanted him to play football with them. Within a couple of minutes, Skye had been hit by the ball, and began to cry. When this happened to one of the boys, Andy simply expected him to be "tough" about it, and to get up and play again. But instead of saying something encouraging and carrying on with the game, Andy ran over to Skye and picked her up. "Never mind," he told her, wiping her tears. "Football is a rough, boy's game, we shouldn't have let you play really. Why don't you go inside and help Granny make dinner instead?" Skye did as she was told.

Several studies were carried out in the 1970s which clearly showed that we treat girls and boys differently from the time they are born:

- Rubin, Provenanzo and Luria (1974) found that parents described their babies using different terms, even though there were no real differences. Baby girls were more likely to be described by their parents as delicate, cute, soft and little; baby boys as strong, hearty and big.
- Smith and Lloyd (1978) showed the same baby to mothers, and found the mothers treated the baby differently depending on whether the researchers told the women that the baby was a girl or a boy.
- Brooks-Gunn and Matthews (1979) showed that other adults also responded differently to babies depending on whether they thought the baby was a girl or a boy.

If you are born a girl, you are more likely than your brothers to be dressed in frilly, impractical clothes and spoken to softly, cuddled when you fall down and given dolls to nurture and pretend food to cook rather than bricks and construction kits to build with. You are more likely than your brothers to be taught the value of communication and negotiation and ~ very importantly ~ of being attractive to others, which will later translate into your spending much more time and money than your brothers on clothes and personal grooming. Your parents and the other adults around you will never have to learn how to do this; most of them will barely be aware of doing it, as this is what they themselves have learned as the 'correct' behaviour from those who came before them. They are also extremely unlikely to question it, even though the way in which we socially construct girls and boys to be different goes on to play a huge part in their experiences of life and of being a woman or a man.*

Your brother, even if he is your twin who your parents perceive is being raised in an equal manner to you, will probably never be taught to be scared of walking outside if it is dark. He can feel safe that, unless he ever goes to prison, his chances of being raped or sexually assaulted are negligible, although, on the other hand, he will have a much higher chance of being mugged than you. He will have a whole variety of reasonably realistic 'superhero' role models to choose from during his childhood, where you will have very few. (Those you do have may be acting more like men than in ways that are strong but also feminine.) If your brother chooses not to have children of his own, his masculinity is unlikely to be questioned, and if he does have children and takes care of them himself, people will think he is amazing even if he is barely competent. He is unlikely to have bad driving, periodic bad moods or bad financial management attributed to his gender. Nobody is ever likely to expect him to realise any of these privileges (although that is not to say that some men don't realise, and work hard to do what they can to change some of these things).

As a little girl, the language you will learn is biased against your gender, with words like "chairman", "man-made" and "manpower" only sometimes, and then clumsily, replaced by more neutral alternatives. The most offensive swear words that exist are slang words for your genitals. Colloquial words relating to men's genitals are, at worst, not ideally suited for conversation with your grandmother. Some of the great historical speeches and quotes ("all men are created equal", "one small step for mankind") can never be changed to reflect the existence of your gender. If you marry, you will be expected to change your name, or, somewhere along the line, to justify why you haven't. You will also either be expected to use a title which denotes whether or not you are available for marriage, or to constantly explain to people who will automatically assume that you are either a "Miss" or Mrs" that there are other options. If you are a heterosexual woman, you may be judged on your ability to 'capture' a man, and may apply the same

* This, and the following two paragraphs are partly based on work by Barry Deutsch, after Peggy McIntosh.

judgement to your own sense of self-worth. If you are a homosexual or bisexual woman, you can expect to be tolerated less than your homosexual or bisexual brothers. If you choose celibacy, you may encounter judgements about your ability (or lack of) to "capture" a man, where your male counterpart will be seen as "playing the field".

There are, then, clear differences between the way we raise girls and boys in our society, and in the attitudes we have people of each gender. However much people argue that women have more equality than before, there are still many facets of life in which this so-called equality is merely an illusion. The point here is not whether there are natural (as opposed to socially constructed) differences between boys and girls; it is the degree to which each gender is respected within society, or whether one has advantages over the other.

In the 1960s, a psychologist called Lawrence Kohlberg carried out a study to assess how good young children are at weighing up moral and ethical dilemmas; at reasoning towards an answer. He concluded that young boys were much better at moral reasoning than young girls, a conclusion which was taken as 'fact' for many years.

In 1982, another psychologist called Carol Gilligan published her updated version of this study. She had given children the same scenario that Kohlberg had and asked them what they thought. Both Kohlberg and Gilligan told the children a story about a man called Heinz, whose wife was very sick, but who could be cured by a drug on sale at the local chemist's shop. In the story, Heinz could not afford the drug, so he stole it, and the children were asked whether they thought he should have stolen the drug.

In Kohlberg's version of the study, the researchers concluded that, because the boys quickly came to a decision which was either "yes" or "no", they were better at moral reasoning than the girls, who were less fixed in their answers. (The researchers didn't really mind whether the answer was "yes" or "no" so much as they wanted the children to decide between one and the other.) Yet, when Gilligan more closely studied the way girls answered the question, she realised that something was going on which Kohlberg had missed.

When the answers the girls gave were analysed, Gilligan realised that they were not less adept at moral reasoning than boys; they simply understood the question differently. Where the boys heard a black and white "maths" question about whether or not a man should steal a drug, and answered accordingly, the girls heard ∼ and viewed ∼ the question in a more fluid manner. They reasoned; maybe Heinz shouldn't have *stolen* the drug, maybe he could have talked to the chemist and negotiated. Maybe the chemist might have been able to do him a deal, or work something out. Some people might think they came up with far more creative solutions to the question than the boys, based on negotiation and communication. Yet because the boys came up with the answer Kohlberg expected, and the girls didn't, he assumed the boys were better at moral reasoning.

Equally, you could argue, Gilligan was looking for an answer which better suited her feminist perspective. It doesn't really matter whose 'answer' we think is right; it matters that we realise that we do still live in a society where there is more than one view, and which generally tends to privilege male ways of thinking and being over female ways of thinking and being. This may be why we have seen the emergence of the high-powered, hard-hearted female executive, and the "ladette" culture, where some young women have taken on the kinds of social behaviours normally exhibited by young men. It is clear from these examples that, in some areas, women have enough equality to have earned the right to behave in the same ways as men. Pregnant women who demand elective cesarean sections may also be seen as exercising the 'right' to deny the natural abilities of their female body; to refuse to be constrained by their biology.

Yet many questions remain, and we still have a lot of gender-related issues to untangle. Are there 'natural' differences between women and men, how do these manifest, and how much does the way we treat young girls affect their gender identity? Should we celebrate winning the right to drink lots of beer and shout lewd things at men, in the way some men feel it is OK to shout lewd things at women? Should we celebrate being able to be ruthless at work, even though a significant number of business experts are now trying to bring about work–life balance or introduce a spiritual dimension into business? Do the things mentioned ∼ and there are many other examples ∼ represent true equality, and, if so, at what cost?

There is, of course, nothing wrong with male ways of thinking and being; they can be very useful and I see no value in throwing all of those things out in favour of a world biased in a different direction. But there may be a case for looking more closely at women's ways of thinking and being in order to try to answer some of these questions, and, if we think there is an imbalance in the world that our daughters are being born into, to find ways to redress this.

Chapter 6

Spiralling into Womanhood

What do young women learn about their bodies as they begin on the journey we call puberty? As they watch television advertisements for "sanitary" products which will hide away their blood from the rest of the world and allow them to carry on "normally"? Do they wonder why the liquid used to demonstrate the absorbency of the products is never red? What does this transmit to them? What do they learn as they read magazines showcasing the bodies of women who are so slim that they may not actually have menstrual periods? As they discover how their changing bodies are viewed by society and learn from those around them whether their femininity is deemed of positive or negative value? As they sit through personal and social development classes and school biology lessons which, for a lot of young women, comprise the majority of the information they will receive, what are they really learning?

> It [menstruation] was a big secret thing, there was only my Mum, Dad and me in the household and it was definitely something that my dad didn't know about.
>
> (Mieke)

> I remember we had a video and also the school nurse did a talk for everybody in the main hall. It all felt very 'matter-of-fact', and not a lot of this is actually a cool thing. It was all very scientific.
>
> (Maggie)

> [I learned] nothing specific, nothing that prepared me for the reality of it. There was this book which was completely useless, it was about a young lad that went on a school trip and when

he came back his voice had completely different and he could see the beauty in architecture and not much about the girls so I don't think I was prepared at all for periods. At school, we were told 'if you find yourself in a mess, or uncomfortable, go and see Mrs Glover'.

(Mieke)

Unlike the women of Joan's generation, young women learn about their bodies earlier than ever before. They begin with pictures which come straight out of medical textbooks, showing cross-sections of women's reproductive systems, quite divorced from the hormones and feelings which conduct the orchestra of their cycles ~ and which may not include the latest knowledge of the clitoris which was discussed in Chapter 3. Indeed, they learn to see the "reproductive system" as one system of the body, apparently working independently of all the others. They see women's organs as motionless diagrams on a page or slide, rather than as wafting, fluid and flowing.

They watch the act of conception in virtual reality; the output of cameras following the journey of semen through women's bodies, with only token reference to the lovemaking that usually precedes this journey. It has always fascinated me that the films I watched at school showed conception beginning from the perspective of the journeying sperm, never from the perspective of the egg, who was also on her own journey ... I wonder how those films would have been different if they were made by some of those ancient menopausal women who had spent a lifetime getting to grips with their creative power ~ if I ever come across a time machine, that would probably be my fantasy mission!

When the idea of hormones is introduced to young girls, it is often in the form of complex graphs showing the varying levels of these hormones during different times of the menstrual cycle. So many young women learn about their menstrual cycle in terms of tissue proliferation and tissue shedding, not in relation to the different feelings they might experience at different times of their cycle, or how their ways of thinking and being might change throughout the month. They may have no concept of the degree to which their minds and souls can influence their cycles. They have no clue that, one day, if they have a male partner, their bodies may decide not to ovulate at "the usual time", which happens to be a day they are away from him, but instead to extend their cycle until they come home a few days later and ovulate on the night they make love.

I asked some of the women I spoke to for any words or phrases they had heard or used to describe menstruation: the following list is of the "top 10" words or phrases in the order of how frequently they were mentioned, and probably speaks for itself:

1. Period
2. On (as in "I'm on")
3. Time of the month
4. The curse
5. On the rag
6. Visitors (which includes "having visitors")
7. Monthly
8. On the blob/blobbing
9. Surfing the crimson wave
10. Waterlogged pitch

Although a few women did mention words which might be seen as more positive, such as "powerful" or "moontime", our culture still seems to have far more words which might be seen as negative, or which are euphemistic, reinforcing the idea that bleeding is not something to be proud of.

I wonder how differently our daughters would see their bodies if, instead of watching films of medicalised cycles and medicalised birth, a busload of grandmothers bearing chocolate cakes came along to talk to them for the afternoon? Would it make a difference if, when dusk came, the girls and the grandmothers moved to sit around a campfire before they were taken to a late-night performance of *The Vagina Monologues* (Ensler 2002)? What about if the handouts were not pictures of inert cross-sectioned bodies, but copies of *Woman: An Intimate Geography* by Angier (1999), whose celebration of female anatomy and physiology includes a glorious feting of the fact that the clitoris is the only organ in the female or male body designed purely for pleasure.

How differently would young women see their bodies and feelings if their teachers did not assume (or, in some cases, were not forced to make the assumption) that they were all heterosexual, but enabled them to explore other possibilities and different kinds of relationship ~ and celibacy? What if another busload of women, each of whom had made a different set of choices in their life, could come along the next day to tell their stories? And what about if they were exposed to a different kind of TV advert; one which showed that, while some women might suddenly decide they want to roller skate during their period, others might choose to relax and rest, either together or alone?

Given the level of educational and medical preamble which most of our daughters now receive about puberty and their menstrual cycles, what do they feel about this when the day arrives? What are their real-life experiences? Duerk (1989) wrote about how wonderful it would be if the day you got your first period your mother took you out for a women's day and your father gave you a red rose. By contrast, Phoebe, who is now in her early thirties, remembers having a period as a completely humiliating experience for herself and her younger sister:

"You went up the stairs to the toilet with a carrier bag. You had to deposit your sanitary towel in the bag and tie a knot [in it]. You then had to inform my father who would be standing at the bottom of the stairs with a second carrier bag which you would then put the first carrier bag with the towel in. He would tie the top and he would put it straight into the [outside] dustbin ... and this would happen when people were there too. So everyone knew about it and you couldn't even change a pad without everyone knowing. Every single time. We would be told to wash our hands before bringing the first bag down then wash again after and so would my father. I dreaded my periods."

"If I got blood on my underwear I used to really panic. We weren't allowed to put them in the wash. I used to try to wash them myself or try to throw them away secretly. My mother would count knickers in the wash. The whole thing was awful. They never said you're dirty or it's dirty but it was such a big trauma. I couldn't wait to get onto tampons because they were allowed to go down the loo. It was definitely a curse. My dad called them your monthlies and it got to the point where you dreaded coming on. I was ashamed."

Nowadays, Phoebe is a confident woman who has realised the implications of the way she was raised to feel about her body and its cycles. She has, as a consequence, chosen to raise her children differently, being incredibly open with both her daughter and son. And some women do seem to reach a point where, despite experiences to the contrary, they spontaneously find their own power and realise that they don't have to feel badly about their bodies; that there are other possibilities.

> *"I started during the school holidays and mum and dad were at work, and I woke up in my pale blue pyjamas and I thought oh my god, I thought shit, and then I thought, ooh, this is it, this is what you're supposed to go and see Mrs Glover about! So I thought, behind the bread bin, that's where my mum keeps her stuff, but there was no sanitary belt, just these things the size of a mattress with loops. They weren't self-adhesive, so I just bunged one in and thought well just wait till my mum comes in. That was the start of it. No indication of when the next one will come."*
>
> (Mieke)

> *"I first started when Mum and Dad were about to go shopping, which is just typical, and I was literally on the loo and I had to call my Mum back. I think Mum came up and rustled around in the cupboard underneath the sink and passed me a sanitary towel and kind of helped me with what to do with it."*
>
> (Olivia)

> *"I remember I started when I was 11 and I was at middle school, and I always remember being so ill prepared and having to go to the nurse and saying 'could I borrow a sanitary towel. And she would say, 'well I don't want it back!'."*
>
> (Maggie)

Social values and beliefs are not only transmitted by our parents and people older than us; our peer group is hugely important to us during puberty and can have a major influence on how we feel about our bodies. During one women's circle, Amelia said:

> *"I went through puberty early, and had large breasts from when I was quite young. And I remember feeling quite embarrassed*

about it. I would cross my arms over them when I walked around, especially at school, where some of the other kids were vicious ... I think if somebody had said at that point that I could've had them chopped off, I would've. In fact, I think I said to our GP could they please do that ... make them smaller ... I was probably about 12."

To which Davina replied:

"Oh, God. I felt I never had breasts, and I was really envious of girls like you who did. So I was probably one of the people who made jokes about it, because I wanted to look like that too ... I never thought about how much that would hurt."

For both Amelia and Davina, this was a point of realisation; a movement onto another level of their spirals. They each realised that their assumptions about what the "other" was thinking may not have been accurate. Once we realise this, once in our lives, we may then begin to question whether we can ever know what someone really means unless we ask them, and we might be far less likely to jump to conclusions. We are so good, as women, at policing other women, and sometimes at accusing other women of trying to police us. It is often not until we sit down and really listen to each other that we can actually take in the diversity of women's lives and understand that we often ~ sometimes inadvertently ~ make each other feel far worse about being women than any man ever could.

How does the journey of puberty feel to a young woman who is on that journey today? If you were a young woman on this journey, what words would you like to hear? What images would you like to see on posters and television? What would be your ideal educational experience? What gifts, if any, would you like to receive?

I wanted something to be different, I wanted people to know but I wasn't quite sure what I wanted them to know. I thought, I'm different now, but it was so throwaway!

(Mieke)

I don't think my parents would really celebrate that sort of thing. It was more that they would brush it under the carpet ~ they're

not the sort of people who would shout about it. I'm sure mum told
dad and that was it ~ they just went off and did their shopping.
(Olivia)

Davis and Leonard (1997) discuss menarche rites; ceremonies which some mothers organise for their daughters' first menstrual period. They may include ritual baths, eating red food, drinking red wine, receiving gifts and, perhaps most importantly, being with a group of other women who share information and stories with them. I didn't have a menarche ceremony, but I spent my thirtieth birthday on a beach in Trinidad. I was with a few women friends, all of whom were older than me. Each of them, as a birthday present, shared some advice with me; things they wished they had known at the age of thirty. This was an incredibly powerful experience, and I can only imagine how much more powerful it would have been if I had been able to experience something similar twenty years before.

Would you like your menarche to be celebrated, or would you like the option of getting on with it yourself without everyone knowing? As a result of her own experience, Phoebe feels the latter option is also important...

"I want my daughter to be able to choose not to tell anybody ...
if that's what she wants."

I like the idea of a menarche ritual, and having a big fuss made of me, but I'm sure it's not what all young women would want. Just as it is unfair to try to impose "one way" of having babies on all women, or "one way" of being a woman or a mother, it also seems unfair to impose one way of greeting puberty on young women. Whether our own experience was of the standard, slightly embarrassed, transmission of medical and sanitary knowledge, or the full-on gala celebration of womanhood, there must be all kinds of other possibilities, or combinations of possibilities, that we haven't yet thought of. While the transmission of societal values to new members of that society is inevitable and important, that is not to say that young people don't have innate understanding and values of their own. Otherwise, we would be suggesting that the souls who were so wise at birth suddenly lose their wisdom when they reach puberty. Some of these souls certainly become more difficult for some of us to understand, but perhaps we could also begin to trust that they know what might be good for them, and incorporate a variety of viewpoints in order to broaden our knowledge together.

Chapter 7

Nature, the Moon and Women's Knowledge

If the Western medical approach to women's bodies is only one way of thinking about our cycles, then what are the others? And if we can find other views, do we try to fit them together in a bigger picture, lay them out as a patchwork of options or choose one solution for everybody? The "one solution for everybody" is what has been offered by Western science and medicine, and the numbers of people who are turning to other approaches suggests that this is not useful as a stand-alone set of ideas. Perhaps, then, the ideal situation would be one where we could look at other approaches and ways of thinking, and then either piece them together into a more integral patchwork of different ideas, or decide which one(s) felt right for us in any given situation.

If we start by thinking about women's cycles and spirals in a general sense, the first issue emerging from women who are seeking to reclaim their femininity from male-based concepts is often that of returning to a more natural (as opposed to medical or technological) approach. Would it benefit us as women to move towards a position where, without necessarily rejecting the benefits of our modern existence and surgical or pharmaceutical help where we felt this was appropriate, we were more in touch with natural cycles and other ways of experiencing the rhythms of our lives?

There are plenty of regular cycles both in humans and the world around us; the daily rhythms of tides, light and darkness, the seasonal changes of weather and food-growth and annual patterns of animal migration and hibernation as well as rainfall, hurricanes, tornadoes and the sun, at the heart of our yearly calendar. And, of course, the monthly rhythm of the lunar cycle, which has long been correlated with the menstrual cycle.

The word moon comes from the Sanskrit word for measurement, and has the same root as the words month, menstrual, menopause and mind

(Grahn 1983; Sjöö and Mor 1987). According to Sjöö and Mor (1987) menstruation also means "moon-change" and "mind-change". Several of the women I talked to while writing this book were in no doubt that their moods, emotions and menstrual cycle are linked with the moon:

"I feel there is something there but I don't have any personal knowledge or experience to actually say yes although I'm sure there is a lot to be said for it ... It just feels right but I don't know how, intuition I suppose."

(Maggie)

"There have been some really key points in my life where all I have wanted to do was sit and be with the moon ... or the ocean. When I broke up with the first love of my life ... I was thirteen ... I went and sat on the beach till the moon came out ... I was freezing, but somehow I needed to wait for the moon. Then I had another really heavy time when I was about twenty-four, and I did a similar thing ... I went and sat on another beach, just before sunrise, and watched the moon set and the sun come up and talked myself through it in my head. Then I kind of picked myself up and got on with it, like it had been washed away and I was beginning again ..."

(Daphne)

"Oh, there's definitely something linked to the full moon. Several years ago I was working with a theatre company and I was doing a lot of festivals working outside. The artistic director said she definitely preferred doing performances when the moon was full because the energy was much higher and stronger. The crowds were much more receptive and our creativity was at it highest ... And that's what got me interested. What I did was, say, don't look at the cycle of the moon, just keep a diary, a creative diary for about five months. When I looked back, I thought 'she's absolutely right', the things I was doing, the really good things, were around about the time of the full moon. That was really fascinating. I think there's something really beautiful about the full moon, the light it can give. I don't monitor it left,

right and centre, but every now and then I'll go outside, it's like sunbathing, just stand there for a few minutes and think it's really nice. I do get a physical feeling, like bright sunlight, like being energised."

(Mieke)

Some people are also convinced from their professional experience that the moon is linked with human behaviour, and words such as lunacy and lunatic have developed from this idea. Some of the nurses who work with people who are mentally ill (whatever that might mean if we had time and space to analyse it) will tell you their behaviour changes. Policemen may tell you that they make more arrests and see more people committing suicide during a full moon. Some of the midwives who work with women choosing natural pregnancy and birth are more reluctant to plan evenings out with their partners and friends at certain times of the lunar cycle because they know from their experience they are more likely to be called out.

Louise Lacy suggested that ancient women may have used the menstrual/moon connection to develop knowledge around natural contraception (Lacy 1974), and many people believe that the moon has even more influence on our cycles than we have previously thought ~ a theory that I must confess I find very attractive. Yet the attractiveness of a theory has little to do with whether that theory is true or false, and this is a really interesting area to look at in relation to knowledge. Some of the people who support this theory are convinced that, among other things, women are potentially fertile when the moon is in the same phase it was at their birth (even if they are menstruating at that time) and that men's sperm counts increase during certain phases of the lunar cycle. One such person is Eugen Jonas, a Catholic psychiatrist whose work and claims are hotly debated on the Internet.

I'm trying very hard as I write this to not sound as if I am believer or a sceptic as far as these theories are concerned, because the fact is I simply don't know, and where I don't know something, I don't want to influence what other people believe. I do find it amazing that, despite all the time that has passed since Aristotle noticed that the ovaries of sea urchins were swollen at the time of full moon, we remain relatively ignorant about the possible effects of the moon on our lives and cycles. Many scientists are among those who disagree about whether these links are 'proven'. We have scientific evidence to show that we were right in thinking that women who live or work together tend to synchronise their menstrual cycles (Coad 2001), but differing opinions on whether there is a scientific basis linking aspects of women's lives such as birth, menstruation or emotional state with the moon and her phases.

Yet it is possible to interpret this in a number of ways, and deciding that something is not true because it has not been 'proven' by science is only one possible view. Some people would argue that, just because something hasn't yet been 'proven' by science doesn't mean it isn't true. Philosophers of science often talk about black swans in relation to this issue: we might create a theory that all adult swans are white, but we can't prove this. This is because, even though we have never seen a black swan, we have to acknowledge that one might turn up tomorrow and disprove the theory. Similarly, a lack of concrete evidence linking the phase of the moon with women's moods or the onset of labour does not necessarily mean there is no connection or correlation between the two.

As another example, no-one has ever conducted a research study to prove that it is helpful to offer women a cold wet cloth to wipe their face with if they become hot and sweaty in labour, yet midwives commonly do this, and would be unlikely to stop if you suggested this might not be useful because it hadn't been scientifically proven. The bottom line is that no-one has ever carried out a research study to find out if this is useful; there are far more important things to spend research money on, and it seems so much like common-sense to us that we have never bothered to check it out.

In the case of the moon, however, there have been a few studies exploring some of the suggested links between the moon and women's cycles, so how can we explain the lack of concrete scientific evidence found in these studies? Those people who believe science to be the best way of gathering knowledge might conclude at this point that there are no links, and anybody who gives their own experiences (and those of others) more weight than science must be deluding themselves. Yet, for other people, there still remain other possibilities. One of these is that modern technology might impact on our experiences. It might be, for instance, that there is a link between women's labours and the moon if women experience pregnancy and the onset of labour naturally, but where they are experiencing medical intervention, this is interfering with their natural cycles and therefore the studies are not showing any links. Even women who choose not to consult doctors or use medical technology when they are pregnant may not have experiences which consistently show a connection; as McLintock (1971) suggested, the abundance of artificial lights in our modern world may interfere with this link in some women.

Yet some people still argue that, in their experience and despite the level of light pollution in many parts of the world, a link exists, so perhaps we haven't carried out the studies rigorously enough. Although we have grown up to believe that science is objective, in reality scientific research is carried out by people who are, by definition, human, with human flaws and biases. Is it possible that we haven't yet carried out a study well designed enough to see the links?

There are numerous examples of medical studies with design flaws that have led to questionable results. For example, a study which set out to find out whether it was better for a woman to give birth to her placenta naturally or for midwives to give a drug and then pull the placenta out suggested that there was less blood loss when this process was 'managed' medically (Prendeville 1988). However, the women who were giving birth to their placenta naturally still experienced other forms of medical intervention, some of which can lead to increased blood loss, and it could be argued that this did not give the natural approach a fair chance (Wickham 1999). Contrary to the results of this study, the many midwives who work with women choosing to birth their placenta naturally do not find themselves continually dealing with women who are losing lots of blood. Midwives, particularly those who work in women's homes, do not like emergency situations, and if we truly believed that giving birth to the placenta naturally was more likely to lead to emergencies, we would be much more uncomfortable where women wanted to do this. Instead, our experience leads us to believe that the natural approach is both safer and more pleasant.

So it could simply be that we haven't looked for the right data in the right way yet, and some people would argue that this might be because scientific studies tend to reflect the prevailing views of the day. If we look at the example of the lunar fertility period, a pragmatist might point out that only a small proportion of women use natural family planning these days, and a sceptic might note that, because there are very few products and no drugs that can be marketed to women who are using these methods, those people who hold the serious money for research are unlikely to see any benefit in researching this claim.

This leaves the individual woman with little choice but to decide whether the possibility of these links may be relevant to her. These were the views of some of the women I talked to (who already used natural family planning) about the possibility of the 'lunar fertile period':

> *I have heard about it, but I don't do anything about it. I probably should ... but I don't know whether it's real or from someone's imagination!*
>
> (Cath)

> *We use natural family planning, and I do use the lunar phase thing, when I heard about it I thought, well, yeah there might not be anything in this, you know, and I know there's no proof, but I don't really care because we do want to wait a while and ... well it's my body, after all, so I have to do what I feel.*
>
> (Tori)

Our society has, historically, tended to see nature and science as opposed to each other. Spretnak (1993) comments that modern culture seems to be in opposition to nature, where the former is ordered and scientific and the latter is unbound and chaotic. Perhaps when Francis Bacon and his colleagues set out to "attack women's secrets", they did so in such a male-centred way that many of those secrets remained hidden from their approach. Our decision now is whether to concur with the scientists that theirs is the only valuable way to find anything out, or begin to look further afield for knowledge about our bodies. We also need to think about whether we will choose to be sceptical about new theories until they are proven (which is a pretty scientific way of thinking in itself) or whether we should welcome new ideas which feel good, and see where our experience of trying out these ideas leads us.

One key study, which has been really important in the debate around knowledge, was carried out by four women (Belenky et al 1997). They talked with women at length and described five different perspectives from which women viewed reality, truth, authority and knowledge. They found a few women, generally the youngest and most deprived, who were "silent"; these women simply did what they were told without feeling that they had a mind or voice of their own. Women tended to move from this position into a place where they listened to the voices of others, and followed what we have come to call "received wisdom". Violet, whose story is told in Chapter 4, would be a good example of a woman in this group; she places more importance on what her doctor tells her than on her own knowledge and experience.

Then there are women who have found their inner voice and intuition, who are described as "subjective knowers". These women may totally reject science and received wisdom as they quest to find themselves and their own knowledge; they may not even want to look at scientific knowledge, preferring their own experiences as data. Several of the women whose experiences because "Joan" expressed this kind of feeling as they talked to me; they had realised their doctors didn't know everything and instead relied on their own and others' experiences to make decisions.

Yet another group seems to have moved through both of the preceding phases into a place where they use reasoned reflection and conscious, deliberate analysis to reach their answers. They may place either their own experience or scientific knowledge at the centre of their knowing (albeit possibly in a sceptical way) and they tend to focus on understanding 'how', rather than understanding 'that'. Finally, there were women who were termed "constructed knowers". These women see all knowledge as constructed by humans, and feel that any knowledge is closely connected with the person who knows it. They feel it important to be really honest in communicating with other people, most are very interested in their own moral and spiritual growth and they have been described as "passionate knowers".

As the authors of this study noted, these categories may not be exhaustive; there may be other ways of knowing that they did not find in their data. As is the case with any model which gets fixed on paper, the reality is not as fixed as it might seem: people may not remain in one category but may move through several, depending on the subject or their mood. With this in mind, it may be more useful to view these categories as different places on moving spirals, where none are seen as right or wrong, better or worse, but all are possible points on a journey.

One of the reasons that Belenky et al's study was so important is that it can help women see where they stand in relation to knowledge; where they are on this spiral, and enable us to think about what some of other positions might look and feel like. Once we understand that it is possible ~ and reasonable ~ to hold one of a number of different views about what the most valuable kind(s) of knowledge might be, it becomes easier to understand why there are conflicts over knowledge, and to see our own place on the spiral in relation to that of other people. Another key finding in this study was that the women highlighted the importance of first-hand experience and gut reactions in knowing; something that, as above, does not always fit with the scientific focus of our society, yet is an important issue for many women.

It may, then, be the case that nobody is *right*, and that the questions raised in this chapter have no correct answer, but are part of a series of possibilities from which we can each choose. Perhaps we each have to come to our own conclusions about what we feel we know, what the truth is for our bodies, whether the moon links with our experiences or has a place in our lives, and where wisdom lies for each of us.

Chapter 8

The Power of Rhythm and Seclusion

Over the last few years, we have learned about a new dis-ease called seasonal affective disorder (SAD), where people find they become depressed during the winter. Given that we live in a society that likes to apportion blame, the blame in this case is generally placed on nature; on the winter itself, or perhaps more accurately on the smaller amount of sunlight that we enjoy during the winter months. The usual cures for this condition include either pharmaceutical or herbal anti-depressants (both of which treat the symptoms rather than the underlying cause) or artificial lights, which "change the terrain" so the body gets more of the summer-type light. But, as with so many other areas, there may be another way, and it is, at least in theory, far simpler.

If we were still living in a world without artificial light, those of us living in non-equatorial regions would have to do more in the summer and less in the winter; we simply would not be able to carry on working after the sun went down. There might be a few things we could do by winter firelight, but we would probably be at home by mid-afternoon and, I suspect, in bed much earlier before it got too cold. By contrast, in the summer months we could stay out later, work longer hours and get more done. Perhaps, then, we were not designed to live life in the way we do today, with little contrast between our waking and sleeping hours in the summer and winter. If this is the case, we may be blaming nature unfairly, when it is our attempts to conquer rather than to follow nature's rhythm that is the real cause.

I mentioned in the last chapter that some of the annual patterns in nature are those of migration and hibernation, and I do wonder whether dis-eases such as SAD may be clues that our efforts to tame nature with innovations such as artificial lighting may not always be in our best interests. Some of us are very attached to spending a couple of weeks away in the sun each year ∼ is this merely a luxury of modern times, or could it be that we are following an instinctive call? Our nomadic ancestors would have sought warmer lands during certain months and, through the modern innovations of the charter flight and the glossy holiday brochure, we do the same. Perhaps the existence of ancient festivals, which occur throughout the year, are pointers to a rhythm of rest, relaxation and celebration which we are now emulating with our foreign holidays, occasional parties and weekend breaks.

There are other patterns of rest which we seem to naturally follow along with our animal relations; we rest from each day by sleeping each night, and since (or perhaps before) Biblical times we have been encouraged to rest one day a week. Our human weeks have not always been seven days long, ranging through history from three to nineteen days (Zerubavel 1985) but Islamic, Jewish and Christian traditions ensured that the seven-day week remained popular until and during the early modern period. Even when, during the French and Russian Revolutions, more "rational" weeks of ten and five days were imposed on the people, these were short-lived ∼ due mostly to public opposition ∼ and the seven-day week returned. Zerubavel (1985: 43) describes the seven-day week as, "the dominant 'beat' of social life."

If we accept that there might be something innate in our needing to rest more in the winter, sleep once a day, relax once a week and celebrate or holiday each year, then it is a fairly small leap to see where the monthly "moon lodge" fits in. The term "moon lodge" is both a noun, describing a place where women go once a month during their period and, perhaps more recently, a verb, describing the act of resting during part or all of a woman's menstrual period. The idea of moon lodging itself is not, for the moment, a theory which we need to wonder about, but something which women have done for centuries. That is, until relatively recent times. A moon lodge might be a tent, tipi or hut and it is a cosy space where women enjoy time together without having to work; even their food being brought to them by others. The best description I have ever read of what it is like to live in a society where moon lodging is the norm, can be found in Diamant's (2002) novel *The Red Tent*:

> *"As the sun set on the new moon when all the women commenced bleeding, they rubbed henna on Rachel's' fingernails and on the soles of her feet. Her eyelids were painted yellow,*

and they slid every bangle, gem and jewel that could be found onto her fingers, toes, ankles and wrists. They covered her head with the finest embroidery and led her into the red tent... The women sang all the welcoming songs to her while Rachel ate date honey and fine wheat-flour cake, made in the three-cornered shape of woman's sex. She drank as much sweet wine as she could hold. Adah rubbed Rachel's' arms and legs, back and abdomen with aromatic oils until she was nearly asleep."

(Diamant 2002: 29)

With this, we can begin to see how the idea of women segregating them-selves during their periods could originally have been a positive aspect of life as a woman in some societies; only more recently having been misin-terpreted as menstruating women being segregated by others because they were perceived as unclean. Although Grahn (1993) found some early societies where women seem to have been isolated by spending the days when they were bleeding sitting in trees, she argues that this was a prac-tical necessity to protect women and their families from animals rather than because they were deemed unclean.

In societies where menstrual blood is seen as a magical substance and menstruating women are seen as wise and intuitive, the dreams and visions of menstruating women are given the same kind of credence that, in our society, is given to scientific research findings (Sjöö and Mor 1987). Where others fear, resent or covet the power that menstruating women hold, their response is to label menstruation as abnormal, menstrual blood as unclean and pre-menstrual and menstruating women as irrational; precisely the ideas our society now holds around this (Grahn 1993; Sjöö and Mor 1987).

Women may well be less rational (and perhaps therefore more intuitive) before and during menstruation than at other times of their cycle, but we don't have to see this as a bad thing. Firstly, I am not suggesting that women cannot be rational during their periods (or during pregnancy, which is a similar situation that I shall come back to in another chapter). While some women might feel more intuitive and have an urge to nest at home during their periods, and more outgoing and rational around the time when they ovulate, this may not be the case for all women. Some may want to rest; others may indeed want to roller-skate. Yet even if a lot of women would choose to rest, if it was totally up to them, I feel sure that women are entirely capable of over-riding their desire to nest and be intuitive; we have had to, in order to live and function in modern society.

We clearly needed to move on from the image of the helpless and dependent middle class Victorian woman, in claiming the rights of women as equal and valuable community members, but it is quite another thing to realise that we are in danger of ending up in a position where we deny difference. If we continue to argue that menstruating women are no different to non-menstruating women, or from men, we are in danger of losing the space that women have to explore what female rites of passage mean for them. There are many theories around the tradition of moon-lodging that we could explore, including whether there are real differences in the ways women think throughout the menstrual cycle.

Whatever your own experience is in this area, the real point is that our modern society tends to place a high value on being rational, and a low value on being intuitive. Which means that, when we hear someone suggest that women are less rational (and more intuitive, although we rarely hear that bit) at certain times of the month, we might feel we are being criticised. Yet if we lived in a society which placed equal value on being rational and being intuitive, or perhaps valued being intuitive even more highly than being rational, the situation might be quite different. What would it be like to live in a society where wandering around feeling different before or during your period did not lead to negative consequences, sarcastic comments or assumptions about the value of your abilities? How would it be to grow up in a society where value was given to your increased ability to be intuitive, rather than taken from your decreased desire to be rational? What would it feel like to be sought out for your intuitive capabilities?

Women who are more intuitive (either generally or at certain times of the month) are not cognitively impaired; they are accessing parts of their brains that others don't reach! If it is true that we only use a small percentage of our brains, then women who are able to access their intuitive brains could be the leading edge in increasing our thinking capacities, or recovering those we have lost. A really sensible society ought to be putting Government money into moon lodges rather than weapons!

How different women's experiences would be today if provision was made to build a beautiful and cosy hotel in every community, where women could check in (for free) during their periods, or when they were pregnant or menopausal. You could go to the hotel knowing that the staff would unobtrusively pamper you and attend to your every need, whether you wanted to hide away in your room or join other women in communal spaces. As soon as you called to say you were on your way, the hotel would send someone (again for free) to your house and place of work to take over all of your work for three or four days. If you didn't feel like driving to the hotel, they would send a courtesy limousine with fat purple cushions in the back for you to lie on. The hotel would have lots of jacuzzi hot tubs and a 24-hour buffet with great food and ample supplies of chocolate, books, art and craft materials, videos and music. All "sanitary protection" (which really does need another name, unless we want to continue seeing our periods as unclean) would be free and the staff would include a well-paid team of post-menopausal women who liked nothing better than to offer kindly, empowering advice and share their own experiences when asked.

The fact that my fantasy hotels are unlikely ever to be built is testimony to how far we have come from a culture which celebrates womanhood, fertility and intuitive ways of knowing in our move towards "rationality for all". Perhaps there are things we could do in order to have this be a reality for our daughters and granddaughters.

One of the questions raised by all this discussion of women's spaces is whether taking a regular monthly break by moon lodging is only for women, or whether men have a similar rhythm of work and rest. I have to confess I have not yet found an answer to this, although I wouldn't want to suggest that only half of humanity should be entitled to this time out in a fantasy hotel! On the other hand, it appears that, in societies which have an established pattern of moon lodging, women who were not menstruating (either because they had not reached puberty or because they had reached menopause) do not moon lodge, so it may be that menstruating women have a specific need for this kind of ritual.

I explained to my partner when I met him that I liked to rest and moon lodge once a month, even if only for a day, or a few hours, and he has always been incredibly supportive of this. He has, though, on a few occasions, asked whether men can moon lodge too. My reply has always been that I would be wholly supportive of him doing this, but that I don't know what a male cycle would look like, and perhaps he should chart this himself and then follow the pattern that emerges. In working towards re-capturing this kind of space for women, I think it might also be quite important to encourage men to figure out what they need in the way of rituals, especially for those men who are increasingly supportive of women's spaces and women's needs.

When I talk about these kinds of issues to different groups of women, one of the first comments that I hear each time is that it may be very well for me to suggest this, but a lot of women can't see how they can fit this into their lives. With more and more people now working at home, or enjoying portfolio careers, there is greater potential for people to alter their working patterns and family lives to build in this kind of time-out, but in case anybody wants to try this but can't see how it would be possible, here are some ideas which have worked for other women...

- A moon lodge does not have to be a three day stay in a luxury hotel ~ it can be a day in bed with a good book, a few hours where you only do things you really feel like doing, a really early night with a relaxation tape the day your period starts or a long bath with lots of bubbles and a "do not disturb" sign on the locked door!
- Some women who have young children trade with their partner or a friend so that each takes the children out on their own for a day in a month and the other can have a day to do whatever they like.
- Other women work with a group of women friends so that this kind of option becomes a reality for everyone.
- While some women genuinely can't take time out, others find it hard to allow themselves to have time off. If there is a chance that the latter is the case for you, you might like to read some of SARK's books.
- One of the questions I ask women at workshops on this topic is: If the idea of moon lodging does not resonate with you at all, then what does? Or, if your period is not the time when you would want to do this, when is? Sometimes, we can only know what we need when we take time to think about our own lives and spirals and what feels like truth to us.

The idea of rhythm and seclusion as important and integral parts of women's spirals is not limited to the menstrual cycle, and these may also be important at other stages of women's ~ and perhaps men's ~ lives. Yet the rhythm of the menstrual spiral is the one that, as women, we live with it for the longest. For some women, this is a time when they 'go inside' in order to regroup and ready themselves for the next loop of their spiral, or take time out to consider where they want to go to next. In the same way that some people make resolutions or set new goals at the beginning of a new seasonal or calendar year, a monthly break allows some women to do the same thing on a more regular basis and helps them learn more about who they are and what is important to them.

Chapter 9

A Time to Dance

You might have noticed that, in the last chapter, I said that moon lodging was a historical fact rather than a theory we needed to wonder about, conveniently skipping over the questions I had previously raised about whether we can 'prove' some of these ideas about women's cycles. Yet, if we return briefly to science (which remains firmly in its place as only one way of knowing) we can find support for some of the ideas about moon lodging and the suggestion that women feel differently at different times of the month. It seems that there could be a biological as well as a historical basis for the idea that women's menstrual spirals naturally create times when we feel like socialising, times to work, dance and play, times when we want to make love and times when we want to rest from the world.

The fact that different levels of hormones flow through our bodies at different stages of the menstrual cycle is well understood and documented ~ and is depicted in some of those charts and graphs from which we learn about our cycles. Most women also know that these hormones influence other physical changes in our bodies during the cycle, such as the position and texture of the cervix and the kinds of mucus we secrete. What we are less often told is that each of these hormones plays a part in influencing our moods, abilities and emotions.

Some of the work in this area was collated by Davis (2000) who wrote a chapter in *Women's Sexual Passages* called "Dancing with our hormones" which, along with the experiences of the women I talked to, inspired some of my thinking for this chapter. Elizabeth lists research which shows that:

- Around the time of ovulation, high levels of oestrogen and testosterone mean that women have more "drive to get things done" (Davis 2000: 48).
- Women do better in athletic competition and rational intelligence tests when their levels of oestrogen are high than at any other time in their menstrual cycle.

- During ovulation, women's sense of smell is at its highest, and is particularly attuned to the aroma of a musky male!
- By contrast, progesterone, the hormone which is higher around the time of menstruation (and is also known as 'the hormone of pregnancy'), causes us to be more reflective.

Many more things are influenced by the menstrual cycle than we might think. Women who suffer from certain illnesses are more likely to experience problems at different times of their cycle. One review of the research in this area found evidence that migraines are more likely when women's oestrogen levels drop, asthma attacks increase in frequency and severity during the premenstrual phase and arthritis may be worse during and just after women's periods (Case and Reid 1998). This review also found evidence that irritable bowel syndrome, acne, diabetes, glaucoma and multiple sclerosis are influenced by the menstrual cycle.

A study of women with breast cancer showed that pre-menopausal women who had surgery for this during the luteal phase (roughly between ovulation and the beginning of their period) had a better chance of survival than women who had surgery during the first part of their cycle (the follicular phase). The difference in this study was quite significant; forty-five per cent of all women who had surgery during the follicular phase were alive ten years later, compared with seventy-five per cent who had surgery at other times of their cycle (Cooper et al 1999). Yet, tragically, some of the women who know this still feel that they have to accept the first date they are offered for this kind of surgery, and there are many others who don't know that it is always a good idea to ask questions about suggested treatments.

Another area that has recently been attracting interest is the question of whether ~ and how ~ women's dreams change during different times of their cycle. Natale et al (2003) showed that the women in their study were in a better mood during ovulation than when they were pre-menstrual and that, although their quality of sleep did not seem to differ during their cycle, their dreams certainly did. Just before ovulation, their dreams were more likely to include positive emotions, male characters, erotic themes and what the authors term 'incongruous' storylines. By contrast, their pre-menstrual dreams were longer and included more negative emotions and female characters.

It is curious to me that, if you search on these kinds of topics, much of the research, including most of that discussed above, focuses on the menstrual cycle in relation to medical issues ~ again underlining the way this is viewed in modern society. The kind of research that looks at positive health (rather than illness), emotions and the practical reality of women's lives is fairly thin on the ground. It is almost as if the menstrual cycle is only really interesting to researchers when it is not normal, or when it influences dis-ease.

Perhaps the most well known dis-ease of the menstrual spiral is the so-called pre-menstrual tension (PMT), which in some circles is known as pre-menstrual syndrome (PMS). A syndrome is defined as "a group of symptoms that collectively indicate or characterize a disease, psychological disorder, or other abnormal condition", again underlining the fact that this experience is viewed in our culture as a medical one. There are over 150,000 English-language web sites on PMS/PMT, the majority of which are sales portals for pharmaceutical drugs, natural remedies or information products about how to treat this condition, and most people would consider that the real experts on PMT are health professionals.

But perhaps there is more to PMS than a group of symptoms and a range of treatment alternatives. In one sense, the fact that PMS is now a recognised medical condition could be seen as a positive step; it wasn't that long ago that this was either ignored, or seen as something which existed only in women's minds. These are the recollections of two women who are now in their eighties:

> *"Well I can tell you we remember it because nobody talked to us about it, we could never consult with anybody about it, well they just had to get on with it because I don't think it was really recognised. We used to feel low and think that's the period coming along. That's something we used to have to fight for ourselves."*
>
> (Rose)

> *"I didn't know what it [PMS] was, not till, well not so long ago. If you felt like that, you didn't tell anybody, you just carried on ... No, I don't think I would have talked to the doctor, (laughing) they'd have thought I was soft."*
>
> (Elsie)

For the past few years, there has been enormous debate around whether PMS is indeed "all in the mind" or a condition brought about by a hormone imbalance, and some people feel very strongly in favour of one or other of these theories. For some women, the fact that PMS is now seen as a medical condition somehow makes it more legitimate as a reason to feel depressed, anxious, tired or experience other symptoms. However, there are huge problems in exploring the psychological aspects of PMT ~ our society still makes massive judgements about psychiatric illness, and if PMT is seen as an inability to cope in any way, then women are well aware they may suffer as a result:

> *"Yeah, I feel crap when I have PMT, I always want to just go to bed and hide. But I don't feel I can ... I work in the city and I have a job with a lot of responsibility ... I don't want my employer to label me as a woman that can't cope, so I get on with it and hide my feelings so people don't, well I don't know why really, I suppose so they don't think I can't cope with the job because I'm a woman and I have these cycles."*
>
> (Caroline)

By contrast, Maggie works for an organisation run by women, where there is a different attitude:

> *"I think how it's really refreshing at work, the times I hear someone say "I'm so sorry I'm pre-menstrual. I'll stop biting your head off soon." I think 'God I can say that ~ fantastic'. And then you hear someone say "It's ok guys, I've come on!" I just think this is really cool because I've never had that before, if I'd said that where I was before, they would have said 'right ... ok' (awkwardly). So it's really refreshing that you can say, 'Sorry I bit your head off, but I'm premenstrual'."*

And Phoebe abhors the fact that some people have a tendency to link any kind of depression or unhappiness to PMT:

> *"I used to deny I ever had PMT. Why are we not allowed to just 'be miserable'? Some men just assume that if you are in a bad*

*mood, it has to be something to do with your menstrual cycle.
So I denied that I had PMT and just used to tell everyone that
I felt miserable. My mum sees it as a weakness, she's very much
like, "get on with life, don't mope around". Hopefully I've taught
my son to be a little bit more sympathetic to his partner."*

With this kind of stigma, no wonder many women have been so keen to
go along with the idea that PMS is caused by a hormonal imbalance.
Indeed, the hormonal imbalance theory does seem to be winning the race
to explain the cause of PMS at present, although new contenders pop up
all the time, often in the shape of nutrients or vitamins which sufferers
are said to lack. Of course, the "PMS cause race" carries large economic
rewards, as the cause determines the treatment. If women are convinced
their PMS is psychological or psychiatric, they may be persuaded to take
anti-depressants or tranquillisers. If it is hormonal then women can be
sold synthetic hormones, and if it is the result of a vitamin or mineral
deficiency, then they will buy supplements. In any of these scenarios,
money will exchange hands.

   While there is little doubt that a few women genuinely suffer from hormone imbalances, nutrient deficiencies and/or altered psychology in the
pre-menstrual period and that many of the treatments offered can make
a big difference to a few women, there is a big element of PMS that is
being all but ignored. We hear little about the social aspects of PMS:

*"You're not allowed to acknowledge it, to pander if you like to
your biological status at any given time because life goes on in
the same pattern and you have to keep on the hamster wheel.
Society just doesn't make allowances for normal fluctuations in
the hormonal state and it's a bit of a joke isn't it really, you
know 'why does it take 3 women with PMS to change a light
bulb', [shouting] 'BECAUSE IT JUST DOES!'. It's not given serious
consideration."*

(Jasmine)

Simply put, those of us who live in the West dwell in a culture which does
not value women's cycles, and which resorts to labelling these differences
as wrong, or pathological, rather than as variations of normal. In 1999,

Hylan et al published the results of a study which had involved tele-phoning over 1000 menstruating women from the UK, US and France to ask them about menstrual symptoms and PMS. They found that up to eighty per cent of these women experienced mood and physical symptoms at certain times in their menstrual cycle. By contrast, women from some Eastern cultures don't actually have the concept of PMS; they do, how-ever, report changes in physical signs and emotional experiences throughout their menstrual cycle. Are Western women's bodies so badly designed that the vast majority of us suffer from menstrual pathology, or could it be that, as Jasmine suggests, part of the problem is that we live in a society that doesn't make allowances for normal feminine fluctuations?

I wonder how closely PMS is related to the expectations that are placed upon us by society and by social norms? If we all stopped trying to be perfect women and actually said and did what we felt like saying and doing (and, perhaps more importantly, stopped saying and doing things we didn't feel like saying and doing), would we report less PMS when researchers telephoned? If we could find ways of working which enabled us to follow our own rhythms and moods, would we be more fulfilled? If we gave up the idea that we have to be calm, collected and happy all of the time, and acknowledged that sometimes we feel differently, would we actually 'suffer' less? Would some of us find our PMS went away if we could allow ourselves to understand that, if we feel like working, we should work, if we feel like going to bed in the afternoon, we should go to bed in the afternoon, and if we feel like roller skating or dancing, we should roller skate or dance?

Although I've focused on PMS here, the same argument might apply to other menstrual symptoms, such as period pain. Unlike many of the organisations who have products to sell, I haven't done a research study to 'prove' that this suggestion works. But I have worked with many women over the last few years who have been looking for ways of redu-cing menstrual symptoms, and I can say from this experience that, when women release the expectations that others have of them, and that they have of themselves, they often find their symptoms reduce or go away completely. Perhaps in another few years people will decide that PMS isn't really a syndrome at all. Perhaps the problem formerly known as PMT will become renamed PME ~ pre-menstrual expectations.

Chapter 10

A Sourcebook of Menstrual Choices

While many people think that the two options for health care are Western medicine and alternative medicine, there is at least one other choice: the wise woman tradition, which is increasingly appealing to women (and men) today. Where Western medicine is based on looking at and treating the symptoms rather than the whole person, and alternative modalities, while looking at the whole person, often promote the idea that we are "bad" and need to go to experts and do special things to "clean up our act", the wise woman tradition attempts to integrate the best of what we have learned from different disciplines, while seeing people as basically whole, healthy and interconnected (Weed 1989). In the wise woman tradition, "good health is flexibility, openness to change, availability to transformation, and groundedness" (Weed 1989: 5).

The wise woman tradition is not about fixing or curing, and it does not see health problems as obstacles. It emphasises wholeness, spirals and transformation; problems become pathways to growth. There are no rules about what will work for an individual, and the individual becomes the source of their own healing and wholeness. Healing is *allowed to happen*, rather than being something that is *done to you*. The wise woman tradition is the only one that embraces the treatment modalities of all of the others, albeit with recognition of the potential for negative effects of some of these treatments on our bodies. Susun Weed is currently one of the main voices of this tradition, and she has developed a 'six-step' tool which can help in deciding what to "do" about a problem, with the order based on the idea of "first doing no harm", i.e. start with the things which have the fewest possible side effects. The steps are as follows.

Step 0: Do nothing (e.g. sleep, meditate, unplug the phone). Susun describes this as "a vital, invisible step" ~ and it is one that we often forget, or don't make time for in our search for "quick fixes", yet sometimes rest is all we need.

Step 1: Collect information (e.g. low-tech diagnosis, reference books, support groups, listening to our own intuition). This is always important before taking action but, again, we sometimes forget this one if we rely on others to tell us what is wrong, rather than collecting lots of information and putting it together.

Step 2: Engage the energy (e.g. prayer, homeopathic remedies, crying, laughter, visualisations, aromatherapy, colour therapy, painting). Energy engagement can be a solitary process, or something that you involve others in, I often think that, once you reach this step, it is important not to forget to keep the previous two steps in mind, for instance by taking time out (step 0) to spend time with your friends, find out what they know and think (step 1) and take time to laugh or cry together (step 2).

Step 3: Nourish and tonify (e.g. herbal teas or vinegars, love, some herbal tinctures, life-style changes, physical activities, moxibustion). This step includes the things most of us know we should do to promote health, such as eating well and taking some exercise, and also some effective but mild toning therapies that not all women will be familiar with.

Step 4: Stimulate/sedate (e.g. hot/cold water, many herbal tinctures, acupuncture, moist massage, alcohol). There may be a risk of dependence upon some of these things if they are over-used, which places them after the first few steps, yet they are not as potent as the treatments in the later steps.

Step 5a: Use supplements (e.g. concentrated vitamins or minerals, special foods like royal jelly or spirulina). Susun differentiates supplements from the nourishing and tonifying substances in step 3, as synthesised or concentrated substances can do more harm than good.

Step 5b: Use drugs (e.g. synthesised pharmaceuticals, whether from the chemist or a doctor, oral and injectable hormones, high dilution homeopathic remedies). Overdose may cause grave injury or death, and side effects may occur.

Step 6: Break and enter (e.g. surgery, colonic treatments, psychoactive drugs, invasive "diagnostic" tests such as mammograms and biopsies). Side effects are inevitable and the treatment may cause permanent injury or death, which is why it is on this list as a last resort.

This tool can be applied to any health or well-being issue, and the information in the rest of this chapter is based loosely around the six steps. The interpretation of what each step means, and the decisions around what belongs where are my own, rather than Susun's. Although she has kindly agreed to let me use the model, any misinterpretation is entirely down to me!

Step 0 has already been explored with the discussions around taking time out during menstruation, or at other times during the menstrual cycle. Some examples of ideas for exploring steps 1–6 are outlined below.

I have used four different symbols throughout the rest of this chapter, so you can see where the information comes from. If the information came from more than one source, then I have included all of the relevant symbols. It is my hope that this key will serve the dual purpose of letting you decide for yourself what is credible information based on your own comfort level, while not leaving anything out just because it has not been scientifically tested, or because it has come my way "on the grapevine". Of course, there will always be other things that I have missed, so this list is by no means inclusive of all possibilities:

- ☽ ~ denotes information which has come from women's experience, and which has worked for at least one woman whom I have talked to.
- ☐ ~ denotes information which came from at least one research study of reasonable quality (and which was not sponsored by the company who manufactures the product being sold!).
- ✳ ~ denotes information which came from at least one research study where the quality could have been better or where the company which sells the product sponsored the research but where the results may still be worth considering.
- ◯ ~ denotes information which has come from another source (e.g. something somebody heard but hasn't tried themselves, a suggestion made in an article but not referenced, a web site which appears to be based on giving information rather than selling

products, or from a letter or email sent to me by someone I haven't talked to personally).

Step 1: Collect information

- Women who want to understand their cycles better, who want to find out more about how they feel at different times of the month or chart physical changes may like to chart their cycles. ☾
- Some woman also recommended keeping a journal or diary, finding that they were sometimes surprised when they realised that they often felt a particular way at the same time of their menstrual cycle each month. ☾

Step 2: Engage the energy

- Some of the ideas which women have used to explore their cycles and any associated issues, such as menstrual pain, pre-menstrual tension (PMT), amenorrhoea (not having periods) or heavy bleeding, include:
  - Painting their feelings, and then seeing what the painting 'says' to them. ☾
  - "Talking it through" with friends. ☾
  - Reading books, such as *The Red Tent* or visiting informational web sites such as www.susunweed.com or www.withwoman.co.uk
  - Using visualisation to understand what is happening in their body and "seeing it better", for example, one woman I knew used the image of a small, gentle, furry bunny in her womb, who carefully stroked and soothed the inside of her womb to relieve any pain or tension during her period. ☾
  - Allowing emotions to come up, and being OK with the emergence of laughter, tears, tension, anger, etc. ☾

Another way of engaging the energy is in thinking about the different pads and alternatives you can use during your period; exploring whether your current option is the best one for you, or whether you are using it out of habit, and might be able to find a better alternative. There are several options to choose from...

- Disposable pads (easy for us but not for the environment!).
- Recyclable (washable) pads (better for the earth but not for some women, as they need to be soaked and washed like cloth nappies).

- Disposable tampons (again, easy for us but carry health risks and take away natural juices as well as menstrual flow).
- Recyclable sponges (used like tampons, again better for the earth and easier than recyclable pads as you can wash them out immediately and reuse them, but some women don't like to use them in public bathrooms).
- Menstrual cups (which are a bit like contraceptive caps and stay in place for a while, they are not for women with latex allergies, and can be messy when you empty them but save lots of hassle with pads etc ~ this is an option that you either love or hate!).

This choice really is a matter of personal taste, but it is interesting that the past few years have seen a significant move away from mass-produced pads and tampons towards alternative products. Some women are concerned about dioxins, which are a by-product of the bleaching process used in mass-produced tampons and pads, while others worry about the millions of pounds of waste from these products. The chemicals used in "super-absorbent" pads are similar to those used in baby's nappies, and can cause irritation to some women, while a few women report that changing from tampons to pads or sponges made a difference to their experience of menstrual pain or discomfort:

> "It made a lot of difference to me when I switched from tampons to towels. I mean, I hated towels when I was younger, I think because I thought real women wore tampons! And I can't even remember why I switched ... I might have read something about how tampons soak up all your normal juices as well as the blood, which didn't sound very nice. Anyway, I did switch, and immediately there was less pain. And I realised that some of the pain I had felt must have come from having this wad of stuff in my vagina ... maybe pressing on nerves and things, I don't know if that's right but it feels like that was it. I would have to be really desperate to use a tampon now ... in fact I can't imagine ever using one again ... in fact as long as there is a toilet roll around I will just wad that up and use that, if I don't have towels with me."
>
> (Li) ☾

Step 3: Nourish and tonify

This step includes:

- Eating foods that nourish you. This may include the foods which are generally considered healthy to promote regular cycles and good digestion or some of the foods which other modalities label as "bad", such as chocolate, or cake. If these are the foods we crave, then perhaps these are the foods we need!
- Light exercise to relieve period pain or PMT, or to regulate periods or bleeding.
- Toning herbal teas, such as red raspberry leaf.
- Love, which can come in many forms...
  - Loving and accepting yourself and not giving yourself a hard time for not wanting to be "in the world" or for being grumpy. ☾
  - Making sure you collect lots of hugs from different people, especially on the days when you need them most. ☾
  - Asking your family to make space for you, whether by going out for the day, making you a nice dinner or playing your favourite game. ☾
  - Arranging a women's evening or day, where you do nothing more complex than lay around on pillows, chat, eat nice food (ideally, take-away or snack foods, that no-one has to prepare), drink your favourite juices or wine (although, strictly speaking, alcohol comes in step 4!), and eat chocolate or cake!
  - Also, if I had a pound for each woman who told me that having an orgasm relieved period pain, PMT and feelings of engorgement, I would be very rich! ☾

Step 4: Stimulate/sedate

While a few of the ideas in the previous steps involved asking other people for help or support, nothing so far has required the assistance of anybody with specific skills. This is the stage at which you may wish to engage the services of someone with specialist knowledge.

- Hot pads or hot water bottles to relieve pain and tension. ☾
- Getting a massage (remedial or therapeutic, perhaps with essential oils ~ although some oils can increase bleeding, so you may want to find out more about this). ☾ ✱

- Acupuncture treatment can help with a number of menstrual problems. ☾ ☐
- Herbal remedies (the following examples are those which seem to work for PMT, and which you might want to do more research on, or talk to a herbalist about):
  - Wild Yam ☾ ○
  - Black Cohosh ☾ ✳
  - St Johns Wort ☾ ☐✳○
  - Agnus Castas ☾ ☐✳○
  - Ginko Biloba ✳○
  - Dong Quai ☾
- Homeopathic remedies (I am not going to list specific remedies here, because they are so dependent on the make-up of the individual, and the specific issue or problem). ☾ ☐
- Some women swear by their TENS (transcutaneous electrical nerve stimulation) machine, which consists of pads which you tape to your back and a transmitter about the size of a mobile phone, which you carry in your pocket or on your belt. The machine sends tiny electrical pulses through the pads; these pulses are said to "distract" the brain from experiencing pain from the nerves near the uterus. TENS is also used for pain in labour, and I know a few midwives who use their machines for their own period pains! ☾ ☐

Step 5a: Use supplements

Bearing in mind that these can sometimes do more harm than good, and need careful research and deliberation, some of the vitamins and supplements which are thought to relieve PMT and/or provide balance (in terms of regularity and/or bleeding) during the menstrual cycle include:

- Vitamin B6 ✳○
- Vitamin E ✳○
- Calcium ✳
- Magnesium ☐○
- Evening primrose oil ☾ ✳
- Calcium carbonate ☐○
- It may also be worth consulting a naturopath at this stage for advice on supplementation and nutrition. ☾ ○

Step 5b: Use drugs

There are a large number of different, over-the-counter and prescription drugs available to relieve period pain and PMT, and to regulate the menstrual cycle. Some of the main categories include:

- Nonsteroidal anti-inflammatory drugs (e.g. ibuprofen).
  - Can reduce inflammation and relieve pain by blocking the body's production of prostaglandins.
  - Common side effects include indigestion, heartburn, nausea, vomiting and diarrhoea. Less commonly, ulcers and bleeding in the stomach, and allergic or skin reactions.
- Painkilling drugs (e.g. paracetamol).
  - Also block prostaglandin production, but in a different way (from the brain rather than at the source of the pain).
  - Side effects are uncommon, but include skin rashes, blood problems and inflammation of the pancreas ~ these usually only occur when people take paracetamol regularly for a long time.
- Hormones (including the contraceptive pill, or contraceptive injections).
  - Can make periods more regular and less painful, and regulate bleeding (the bleeding experienced by women on the pill is not a period per se, but a "withdrawal bleed").
  - Common side effects include weight gain, headaches, breast tenderness, nausea/vomiting and fluid retention. Less common (but more scary) side effects include blood clots, depression, skin problems and increased risk of breast cancer, strokes and heart attacks.

Step 6: Break and enter

This step includes some of the tools which Western doctors use to investigate and treat problems with the menstrual cycle, all of which carry risks, implications and possible knock-on effects. Examples include:

- Blood tests, which can check for anaemia and other health problems that may have an impact on your menstrual cycle. They can also measure the levels of your hormones at certain times of your menstrual cycle; the results may lead to the recommendation of drugs or further treatment in this category, so women may want to consider the implications of these.

- Pelvic/vaginal examination, which may be done with the fingers and/or a speculum. Enables the practitioner to see and feel whether any of the organs are enlarged; this can help detect fibroids, endometriosis or polyps and swabs or tissue samples can be taken. Can be uncomfortable or painful (emotionally as well as physically), and can occasionally introduce infection.
- Intra-uterine devices, which are also used as contraceptives. Some of the newer versions of these contain hormones and can make a woman's periods lighter and less painful, although others can increase both pain and bleeding. Side effects include all of those of hormones, plus the risk of physical damage, and reduced fertility.
- Ultrasound, which enables a doctor to view your uterus, fallopian tubes and ovaries to find out whether you have a physical abnormality or blockage. The side effects of ultrasound have not been well-researched (see Chapter 11) and this may also lead to recommendations for further treatment in this category.
- Surgery, which carries serious risks (further increased where general anaesthetic is used) and includes:
  - Hysteroscopy, where a camera is passed through a woman's vagina and into her womb. The lining of the womb (endometrium) can then be inspected by the doctor, who may also want to take tissue samples to check for abnormalities.
  - Laparoscopy, where a camera is inserted through an incision in the woman's abdomen allowing the doctor to visualise the organs. Commonly used to diagnose endometriosis, which may cause irregular and very painful bleeding.
  - Dilatation and Curettage ("D and C") where, under anaesthetic, a doctor will use a surgical instrument to scrape the lining of a woman's womb out. This may be suggested for heavy or painful periods. Recovery can be uncomfortable, and damage may be done to the uterus.
  - Endometrial Ablation, which removes about 5–6 millimetres of the lining of the uterus using heat from an electric current, a laser, cryotherapy (extreme cold) or microwaves. It is an alternative to hysterectomy (below) and stops periods altogether, although some women find their periods return and become heavier than before.
  - Hysterectomy, or removal of the uterus, is sometimes recommended for serious menstrual problems (e.g. excessively heavy periods or

cancer), in a woman who either feels she has completed her family, is sure she does not want (or is not able to have) children, or feels it is the only option left. Carries serious potential side effects and women take a long time to recover.

Given the potential ramifications of some of the options towards the end of these lists, no wonder women are increasingly choosing the wise woman approach and trying the simpler, less hazardous, self-directed options first in the hope that they may not have to resort to the later choices! It's curious, though, to notice that, if you look at the changes in the symbols throughout the list, far more research has been carried out on the later, more complex and risky options than on the simple ones...

Chapter 11

The Journey of Pregnancy

While the hopes, dreams and fears of pregnant women have probably changed little over time, some of the experiences that characterise the journey of pregnancy today couldn't be more different from the experiences that characterised the journey of pregnancy for our grandmothers and great-grandmothers.

For a start, we find out that we are pregnant far sooner than our grandmothers did ~ and in different ways. While some women have always had the ability to intuitively know when they are pregnant, our grandmothers usually had to wait until they had missed a couple of periods or had some other concrete sign to be really sure that they were expecting a baby. Where the realisation that they were pregnant might then have dawned slowly on our grandmothers, for us the confirmation comes quickly, in more ways than one. The location of this realisation may also be different. I don't know whereabouts in their homes most of our grandmothers found out they were pregnant, but I suspect it was probably not in the toilet. But that is where many women discover they are pregnant today, as they sit on the side of the bath or lean on the sink while they wait to see if the little line in the pregnancy test turns blue.

Modern pregnancy tests can be carried out within days of conception, before any physical signs such as breast changes might be noticeable. You can find out that a baby is nestling into your womb almost while it is happening ~ a bit like the flight arrival boards at airports that are constantly updated to herald the arrival of your friends as their plane touches down on the runway and then taxis to the gate. The test itself takes only three minutes, paralleling other aspects of our instant society ~ fast food, e-mail and systems for transferring and withdrawing money at the press of a button. All of these things are terribly convenient, and none are inherently bad, but it is easy to forget how much life has changed in a short space of time, and we rarely think about the impact these changes might have on our experiences of journeys such as pregnancy.

Having found out that they are pregnant, the next thing most women do is go and see a doctor, despite the fact that doctors are specialists in ill-health, while pregnancy is a totally normal, natural and generally healthy journey. Within weeks of conception, the vast majority of women also find themselves watching an image of a tiny person floating inside their womb courtesy of a machine that can look inside their body. Our grandmothers relied on their intuitive connections with their bodies and babies, and learned patience as they waited to see those babies, not knowing what the baby's gender, size, shape or state of health would be. We no longer need to do this ~ we have machines and technicians which can give us the answers.

I am not, by the way, criticising those women who do these things; these are the very things you are expected to do in our society when you become pregnant. From the very first weeks of being mothers-to-be, we behave like "good girls", doing what we are expected and told to do, and we step on to the pregnancy conveyor belt, often without thinking about the implications. Yet there are both advantages and disadvantages to the current 'medicalisation' of pregnancy and the machines and tests used to assess our health and that of our unborn babies.

For example, the ultrasound machine, with the help of its operator, will churn out a date on which the tiny person might be born. Even if the dates of the woman's cycle have already led to the calculation of a date, the machine's date will usually be seen as more accurate ~ although there is no good evidence that this is actually the case. There is a 33–1 chance that this particular date will be wrong, but this should be the least of our worries. The date, decided so early on in pregnancy, will determine all sorts of things later on, including the accuracy of any other tests we may decide to have to assess the health and well being of our babies. It may also lead to us being told that the birth of our baby needs to be induced, if the baby has not been born within the time frame that has come to be seen as the "normal" length of pregnancy.

I wonder how many women would ask more questions about these things if they knew that the "normal" length of pregnancy (generally considered to be two hundred and eighty days) had been decided on the basis of the experience of only one hundred women who lived and gave birth to their babies several centuries ago (Baskett and Nagele 2000)? Despite the fact that several researchers have suggested that this dating system should be revised (Bergsjo et al 1990; Mittendorf et al 1990; Rosser 2000), such revision has not taken place in mainstream medicine and the research which raises questions in this area has been all but ignored by most professionals.

We trust these machines to tell us if our baby is well and healthy. Yet they are nowhere near infallible. Hundreds of women terminate their pregnancies because an ultrasound scan found their baby to have a problem, disability or abnormality, only to make the horrific discovery afterwards that their baby was actually perfectly normal. Other women are lulled into a false sense of security because the machine and its operator suggested their baby was healthy, and then find out at the end of their labour that they are the parents of a baby who has extra needs ~ for which, following the 'reassurance' of the test results, they are totally unprepared. It is not only these scenarios which are anxiety provoking; many of the women who spend time waiting for any test results during pregnancy find that these periods of waiting are much less enjoyable than the times during their pregnancy journey when they are not waiting to hear "what the tests say".

Then there is the fascinating question of the safety of ultrasound. This technology, originally intended only for women who were experiencing problems (where it can be of huge benefit on an individual basis) is now applied to all women on a routine basis. But whether or not you believe ultrasound is safe depends on how you feel safety is assured. There are a number of doctors who have been outspoken about the safety of ultrasound, claiming that there are millions of perfectly healthy people walking around who were exposed to ultrasound in utero and no apparent reason to think that it has harmed them in any way. Yet some people believe it is not acceptable to claim that ultrasound (or any other technology) is safe just because it has not been "proven" unsafe ~ especially when no one has actually carried out the kind of research which would enable an accurate assessment of safety.

A few studies have suggested that ultrasound may cause problems; these problems tend to be behavioural and subtle, rather than physical and obvious. Dyslexia is one example of this; a link has been found between ultrasound and dyslexia, although no clinical trials have been carried out to see whether this correlation is significant (Beech and Robinson 1994). Yet people with dyslexia do walk around and function quite normally, in contrast to people who have been physically damaged by 'advances' like thalidomide. If we do not conduct studies which are specifically looking for subtle and behavioural differences in people who have been exposed to ultrasound in the womb, we are very likely to miss them.

The whole situation begs a number of questions. Do we choose to believe that a technology is safe unless very obvious evidence jumps out at us (as in the case of thalidomide) that it is not? Should we become more sceptical of new technologies (as people seem to be at the moment in the case of genetically modified food) until we believe for ourselves that they have been proven safe? Do those who introduce new technologies have a moral obligation to set up appropriate independent studies to assess their safety before they are unleashed on large populations of people?

These questions are particularly pertinent when we consider that technologies such as ultrasound massively alter the focus of pregnancy in modern times, especially if, like Emma, you thought pregnancy would be a soft and pleasant journey:

> "I had this idea, you know, that I'd sit around, like in dungarees and sort of sit in the garden [laughs] and bloom. You're supposed to bloom, aren't you ... But it wasn't like that at all. I sort of wish it had been, I wish I could go back and do it again."

Instead of sitting around and blooming in her garden, Emma spent a fair amount of time waiting on test results and worrying because her baby did not seem to be growing at the usual rate:

> "They did all these things to find out how the baby was growing, they didn't think she was growing well enough. At one point I was having scans about every week. Then I realised that they couldn't do anything about it anyway, they couldn't make her grow more whatever they did. I wondered why I had bothered, but you want to do everything you can, don't you?"

Emma is just over five feet tall, and her partner is five feet six. Together, they created a perfectly healthy baby girl, who weighed just under six pounds at birth and who, when you look at the photos taken just after the birth, seems to be just the right size for Emma's arms.

In Chapter 8, I talked about how our menstrual cycles seem to create for us times when we are rational and times when we are more intuitive. Many midwives, especially those who try and help women to experience the sacredness of pregnancy, will tell you they believe pregnancy is a time where women are more intuitive than rational. Yet the systems of care offered to us during pregnancy seem to force the need to be more rational, as we have to pick our way through the maze of screening tests on offer and the sometimes horrendous decisions that we need to make. No wonder so many women find it simpler to go with the flow and do what they are told. This then makes it so much more tragic that it is the women who have to spend the rest of their lives living with the decisions which were sometimes made for them.

> *"I wish I'd known then what I knew now, about the risks of some of the things they do. I wouldn't have done half of what I did do. I might not even have gone to the clinics."*
>
> (Tracie)

Given that so many women are shocked or dismayed by what happens once they embark on their pregnancy journey, coupled with the argument that pregnancy is a time where you may not want to be over-rational about weighing up these choices, I wonder if one answer is to try to find ways of helping women find out about and think through the different options before they become pregnant. That may be the one way we could help individual women decide whether they truly want all of the technology that modern science can offer on a routine basis or whether they want to work towards reclaiming pregnancy as a sacred, personal space and use technology only when it feels appropriate for them. This is not to say that the use of technology during pregnancy means it cannot be sacred. But women who are bombarded with choices or, perhaps worse, who find themselves subject to routines without regard for their individual needs, may not find their journey feels as sacred to them as it could.

Every woman deserves to have her individual journey honoured by those around her, and this is the subject of the next chapter. Many people are working to try to enable more women to become informed about the options and for them to be able to choose to experience pregnancy as a sacred space, with or without modern technology. There are midwives who will wholeheartedly support and be with women who want their pregnancy to be more sacrosanct than is the modern norm. More and more women are beginning to rediscover what the journey of pregnancy can mean in a context that embraces and values the spiritual and personal aspects of this journey. There are few women who want to reject all of the technologies which have been developed, but there are many women who would like to step off the conveyor belt and use those technologies appropriately for their individual journey. Meanwhile, these women may choose to sit in their gardens and bloom, enjoy the intuitive nature of their minds during this time and to flow through their journey with a greater sense of the enjoyment that this spiral can bring.

Chapter 12

Childbirth Choices

Not too long ago, a new mother was interviewed on British television by a well-known and likeable female chat show presenter. When the woman told the presenter that she had chosen to give birth at home, the presenter remarked upon how brave she felt the woman was. By contrast, other people believe it is the women who choose hospital birth (or, perhaps more accurately in some cases, do not actively choose the place where their baby will be born at all, but who follow the modern trend to give birth in hospital) who are brave. Unless women have one of a very small number of serious medical conditions which render hospital birth safer, they and their babies are more likely to be subject to unnecessary interventions, suffer problems, contract an infection or have an operative birth if they go to hospital (Tew 1985).

However, the majority of women do not consider giving birth at home or, if they do, are talked out of this idea very quickly during their first interactions with health care providers. Although most women know that some women do give birth at home, most, like the nice television presenter, assume that hospital is the best place to give birth and that professionals know more than they do about these things. This does not only apply to the place of birth decision; women tend to follow social norms and the generic advice handed out by professionals.

Some of the women whose stories became "Violet" and "Joan" (in Chapter 4) used interesting language when they talked. They spoke of "falling" pregnant, as if it were something that happened to their bodies without their having much control over the process of creation. They talked, as some medical professionals still do today, not of home birth, but of home "confinement", as if birth was something involving incarceration. Few women today experience childbirth as a sacred space and a time of incredible growth. Yet it can be both of those things, and much, much more.

Every woman is totally unique. We can each be assured that there is no-one else anywhere who is quite like us. Our individual bodies, minds and spirits have grown and developed over our life spirals, making every woman in the world an original and special individual. Our bodies each have their own special abilities, our minds and spirits are capable of many things, and we have needs which relate to our own make-up; none of which are quite the same as anybody else's. So why should women be treated as if we were on a production line, with the same needs and characteristics as everybody else? Although there are many midwives who offer individualised, community-based care to the women they serve, most women still end up experiencing maternity care within a system, where routines and generalised protocols are often necessary in order to organise the functioning of bureaucracy, institutions and staff.

Women have been having babies since the beginning of time, and it is only in the last few decades that doctors and institutions have become involved with the process. While many professionals believe they are intervening in the birth process 'for the best', research consistently shows that this is not the case; that low-tech, high-touch midwifery care carried out in women's own communities and homes still gives women the best chance of having a safe and satisfying birth. Hospital obstetric care has led to the creation of routines which, in some areas, are imposed upon all women, regardless of need, and which often lead to problems.

Another effect of the movement of birth into the realms of medicine and hospitals is that women have begun to doubt their bodies' ability to give birth. While women have been having babies successfully for thousands of years, women today do not always learn to trust their body. Instead, they fear the birth process, seeing it as something which they need to fight, rather than a rite of passage which marks their journey into motherhood. Midwives know that women's bodies work, and they work hard to enable women to trust their own bodies, and to enjoy their pregnancy and birth as a remarkable and special time for them, their partner, their family, and their new baby.

Although it may seem obvious that when I talk about 'individualised care', we mean care that is tailored to the individual's needs, this involves several different aspects. For those who are trying to make this a reality for every woman, individualised care means that:

- The woman's needs and individuality should be taken into account at all times, and her own body knowledge, intuition and wishes respected.
- The woman should be at the centre of the experience, and have the final say in any and every decision.
- Care providers should have no 'routines' which are applied to all the women she or he serves. Although care providers may have general patterns ~ for instance the times during pregnancy in which they visit or see women ~ these patterns should be flexible and open to change.
- In particular, care providers should not impose routine interventions upon women. Each woman needs to make an informed choice about any intervention in pregnancy and birth, by weighing up the evidence and deciding what is best for her.
- Care during childbirth should be an empowering and positive experience, where women are enabled to grow, to feel good about their bodies, and to begin their life as new mothers with the knowledge that they are special and worthy of their new role.
- Babies also need to be respected as individuals, with consciousness and a unique character. They should be treated gently, kindly and with the utmost respect at all times.
- The needs of the woman's partner and family are also important. For instance, if the woman has other children, their needs should be taken into account and they should be welcome to attend the birth if the woman wishes.

Individualised care is about respect, dignity and empowerment. Sadly, many women do not experience these things. The care provider who offers an individualised experience will see each woman as a unique and special person, who has knowledge about her body and her needs, and will support women in meeting those needs during their experience of pregnancy and birth. While this kind of treatment is very different from what some women experience, it still remains possible:

"I felt so good about my pregnancy with Jane as my midwife. She made me feel like I was the first woman ever to have a

baby. I mean, I thought that too, but she made me feel really special. She helped me feel really confident about my body and I felt like, if she was so sure I could do it, then maybe I could!" And I did!

(Corinne)

Just knowing the person who will be with you during the journey of birth is enough for some women, as Sam discovered:

"I wanted... no, I think I needed... to feel like I was more than a number in a hospital. I had issues, from when I was younger, and I didn't want to not know who would be with me when I was in labour ... Or be at the mercy of machines ... It was so important to me to know the person I would be with, to be able to talk to her about what I needed, and what I didn't want."

(Sam)

These women are not alone in feeling this way. The *Know Your Midwife* study (Flint et al 1989) showed that women who experienced continuity of support and care from a midwife had better outcomes than women who received standard care. Women who knew their midwife felt better able to communicate with her and had fewer anxieties and interventions. This scheme appeared to benefit women 'in almost every aspect investigated'. Similarly, the 'One-to-One' study (McCourt and Page 1996) demonstrated that women who were treated individually needed less pain relief, received fewer episiotomies* and less continuous electronic fetal monitoring in labour. They were also less likely to have their labour speeded up with drugs, and more likely to have a vaginal birth.

Corinne and Sam both gave birth at home, and felt that the individualised care they received gave them and their babies the best possible start in their new life together. Avril experienced medicalised care for one of her births, and found that this did not meet her needs or expectations,

---

* An episiotomy is a cut into a woman's birth canal which supposedly makes it easier for the baby to be born. It can also cause a lot of pain and other problems for women and should never be carried out routinely.

so chose to get to know a midwife who would be with her in the hospital the next time around:

> "When I was pregnant with my third baby (a little girl), I had opted for a home birth with a team of midwives. The pregnancy went well, but at thirty-four weeks she was in a breech position and was still in that position at thirty-six weeks."
>
> "I asked if the doctor would try and turn her by external version, as I really wanted a normal birth at home. I was told that they didn't practice this and I was advised to have my baby at the hospital."
>
> "Being told this as you can imagine was devastating for me as I had already planned for my labour. What I didn't then realise was the full impact of what the doctors had planned for me. I later discovered that not only did they wish me to have the baby at the hospital, they also planned that once the baby was imminent, I would be moved to the operating room. I would lie on a bed with my legs up in stirrups and try and push the baby out, or failing that they would try and pull her out. They suggested that I should have an epidural for this, something I hadn't even considered, as I hadn't needed any pain relief with my previous two labours."
>
> "When the big day arrived I was about to go to bed when my waters broke. From then I laboured quickly and by the time I got to hospital I was having lots of strong contractions. On arrival I was examined and found to be eight centimetres dilated, but she had also changed position and they decided I needed a cesarean. By this time I must have seen about six different faces, each hurrying around doing their own thing and, whilst each was very friendly, I didn't feel that anyone was connecting with me. I was very frightened and my husband was very frightened. Medically all went well, but I knew I didn't want to ever experience this type of birth again."
>
> "Two years later I was pregnant again ~ and wiser. I chose to go to hospital but definitely wanted a midwife I knew and respected to be present at the birth. I really needed her to listen to me and connect with me. I wanted to trust what I was being advised. I didn't want to be bulldozed as I felt I had been previously."

"Before I went into labour we discussed fully our needs and expectations of each other. I felt secure with this arrangement and very much enjoyed my pregnancy."

"During the last three days of pregnancy I kept feeling that I was about to go into labour and that the baby would probably arrive a little earlier than expected. I kept in contact with my midwife during this time and was happy that all the necessary plans had been made. When I finally started labouring we both agreed that I should go straight into hospital due to my previous quick labours. Myself, my husband and my sister met her there. We all seemed to settle very quickly. It was nice that all the important issues had been discussed and that my labour was not interrupted by a continuous barrage of questions, particularly as I did labour very quickly and therefore didn't have much time to get into the swing of labour."

"Having a midwife who I knew and trusted made an enormous difference to my experience. I feel all women deserve to have this opportunity. By the way ~ our third girl was born safely and with no hitches."

Some midwives and doctors strive to offer individualised care because of the unique philosophy they have on life and birth. They believe that the aspects mentioned in the list above are so important that they go out of their way to make sure that women receive care which meets their needs. They actively strive to make women's experiences sacred.

But do we have to choose between 'sacred' experiences and 'safe' experiences? Happily, over the last few years, research has consistently shown that we can have both. In 1989, a group of British researchers undertook a mammoth task in compiling all of the research which existed in the areas of pregnancy and childbirth (Chalmers et al 1989). The book is called *Effective Care in Pregnancy and Childbirth* and is known in some circles as the 'Midwife's Bible'. In the back of this book they listed a number of "forms of care that should be abandoned in the light of the available evidence". This list included the following:

- Failing to involve women in decisions about their care.
- Failing to provide continuity of care during pregnancy and childbirth.

- Involving doctors in the care of all women during pregnancy.
- Insisting on universal institutional confinement (hospital birth for all).

More than fifteen years on, these things are still, sadly, the reality of the childbirth spiral for many women, despite the fact that individualised care has been shown by a large number of research studies to be effective and positive for women and their babies. One American study (Rooks et al 1992), which compared women who went to birth centres for their pregnancy, birth and postnatal care with women who went to doctors' offices and hospitals, found that over ninety-nine per cent of the women who had birth centres said they would recommend this kind of experience to their friends. Clearly, women prefer individualised care which respects the sacredness of their journey when they have a chance to experience this. Which makes it all the more tragic that so many women don't even know that they have these choices.

Chapter 13

The Sensations of Labour and Birth

One of the reasons women tend to choose hospitals for the birth of their baby may be because of the pain relief which is on offer there. It is a commonly held belief in our modern culture that labour and birth is a painful journey and, indeed, many women find this journey so painful that they choose to have the lower half of their body anaesthetised in order to cope with it. But other women experience birth without any pain, and some women even experience intensely joyful sensations. How can this difference be explained and, perhaps more importantly, is it only a select few women who can experience birth with joy rather than pain, or is this a secret that more of us could discover?

Firstly, a quick look at some of the historical aspects of pain will give us a few clues as to why so many women in the West today see birth as painful, pain as negative, and epidurals as the best thing since sliced bread. Several hundred years ago, the idea that pain was a form of punishment grew into a cultural belief. As a result of this, people weren't able to alleviate their own pain. Instead, pain had to be "destroyed through the intervention of a priest, politician or physician" (Illich 1990: 155). We can see from this that we have a fairly long-held view that pain is a 'bad' thing, alongside the idea that it can only be taken away from us by others.

Even today, pain is viewed pretty negatively. Most of us don't welcome pain; we seek to dull it, whether with pharmaceutical drugs or home remedies, such as herbal packs, ice or hot baths. Some of my osteopath friends believe that backache (as just one example) is the body's way of telling a person to rest. They believe that resting is one of the best things you can do when you have backache, and that taking painkillers is not a good idea. Their rationale for this seems very logical to me; they suggest that painkillers only allow us to stress our body further by dulling the pain and enabling our bodies to move in ways that can worsen the injury. Of course, we live in a culture where we are expected to take painkillers and "get on with things", and people are sometimes very surprised if we choose not to do this. I am not a big fan of painkillers and have experienced a few negative comments from people over the years who could not understand why I preferred to remain in pain rather than pop a pill, or perhaps go to bed in the middle of the day because I had a headache.

There is then the matter of the differing interpretations and beliefs around the Biblical story of Eve, Adam and the apple that led to pain in labour for both of them. There are endless arguments about what this story actually means, which have led variously to debates about patriarchal oppression of women and whether women have the right to pain relief in labour. Certainly the Christian church held fast for many years over the idea that women deserved to suffer in labour and, perhaps partially as a result of this, pain relief in labour was not legitimised until Queen Victoria used chloroform in 1847 (Arms 1994; Vincent Priya 1992). However, it took no more than a few decades for pain relief to become a normal part of the childbirth experience, albeit still mostly under the control of doctors. Indeed, pain relief remains one of the main functions of doctors involved in birth.

So we can say that we have some fairly strong historical influences on our beliefs about pain, and this becomes even more apparent when we look at how women experience the sensations of labour in other cultures. Several research studies have been carried out to compare the sensations experienced by women from different cultures during labour and birth. In one study, Anglo women perceived the greatest amount of pain, followed by East Indian women and Hutterite women, with Ukranian women perceiving pain least of all (Morse and Park 1988). In another, Middle Eastern women displayed more pain behaviour and rated their pain more highly than Western women (Weisenberg and Caspi 1989). Harrison (1991) then showed that Bedouin women did experience pain but did not display pain behaviours, while Pathanapong (1990) found that Thai women expressed their pain very subtly.

These results suggest two things. Firstly, it seems that women from different cultures do seem to experience different levels of pain during their birthing journey. But it also seems that, even where women may be experiencing similar sensations in labour (although we can never know for sure what somebody else is feeling), women from different cultures define those sensations differently.

Dick Read (1942) was one of the first people who realised that labour pain might arise from socially induced expectations, and that labour itself was not necessarily a painful process. These ideas were confirmed in Green's (1993) study of English women. She found that the women who had a lot of anxiety about the pain they might experience during birth were more likely to have negative birth experiences than the women who were less anxious about the potential pain they might experience. Anxiety about the pain of labour was also a strong predictor of lack of satisfaction with the birth, and poor emotional well-being postnatally. In general, women tended to get what they expected.

Would we be better off, then, if we expected labour and birth to be joyful experiences? If we could find ways to welcome the challenge of labour and birth, understanding that it would be hard work but also intensely rewarding? Nature does, after all, give us the most amazing natural pain relief in the form of endorphins ～ 'happy hormones' which are created by the body in response to hard work and which give people such a high after hard exercise. In fact, if you look at pictures of athletes who have just won races, their faces look remarkably similar to the faces of women who have just given birth. I noticed this especially when I met up with my friend Lorna as she finished her first London marathon; her pupils were hugely dilated and, when I suggested that she might like to change into a clean, dry t-shirt, she simply put her arms up into their air like a child would, wordlessly asking me to do it for her. She was in an altered state, a very happy state, and a state I had seen many women in before ～ when they were giving birth*.

I don't want this to sound like I am suggesting that all women should avoid drugs during labour and birth; I think it is fabulous that women have the choice of being able to use drugs if this is the right choice for them. But this is yet another instance where we hear little about the normalcy

---

* There has been quite a debate in midwifery circles about whether it is accurate to compare labouring women with marathon runners ～ some people are convinced this is an accurate comparison, while others are equally convinced that it is not. You will find an article on www.withwoman.co.uk written by Lorna, who has done both at least twice!

and positive side of a female rite of passage because this perspective is drowned out by our cultural beliefs about pain being bad, and that we need technologies and drugs to help us cope with it.

People who are interested in this area talk about the need to "surrender" to the sensations of labour rather than being engulfed by them. Ina May Gaskin writes about her experience of being a midwife in an intentional community in Tennessee where "women and girls have little or no fear of childbirth" (Gaskin 2003: xi) She talks about how birth can be painless, even orgasmic, for some women, and how it could be like this for many more. Other midwives echo the idea that women who go into labour and birth knowing that they can do this, and can get over the fear that our culture seems to have of birth, generally begin their lives as mothers knowing that the can do anything:

> *"Labour is a woman-building enterprise! And, if you kill the pain, you kill the joy as well."*
>
> (Sunita)

Women, too, talk about the benefits of "doing it themselves":

> *"My daughter's birth was almost painless ... I had to concentrate on the contractions ... they were massive toward the end, but I never felt what I would call pain ... As she was born, I felt, well just amazing ... more amazing than ... well, I can't even really describe it ... Yeah, I'd do it again just for that bit!"*
>
> (Tina)

> *"Afterwards, I felt quite pissed off ... that I could have had an epidural, if I'd listened to the midwife who said that'd be a good idea. I would have missed so much."*
>
> (Vicky)

Whatever advantages pain relief in labour carries for women, it also carries the major disadvantage (among other side effects) of preventing us from finding out how strong we really are. If we viewed the labour and birth spirals as work, rather than pain, would we approach them differently? I have deliberately used the word "sensations" rather than "pain" in the title of this chapter, because as soon as we use the word pain, it brings up all of the emotional and social baggage which is linked to this word in our minds. Likewise, the word "contraction", as used to refer to the action of a woman's womb in labour, can bring to mind words like spasm, tightening and convulsion ~ none of which feel particularly pleasant or sacred to me. Because of this, Ina May Gaskin and her colleagues in Tennessee use the word "rush" instead (Gaskin 1990). While I have to confess I have never become entirely comfortable using the word "rush", perhaps because of my own cultural baggage, I definitely feel we could develop some more woman-friendly words around labour and birth and the sensations that they bring.

There is little doubt we have reached a point in our social and cultural development where we have a tendency to medicate lots of aspects of our lives. There are drugs or treatments available for almost everything that causes us any kind of pain. We learn that pain is bad, and that it can and should be removed from our lives. Yet, if women didn't experience sensations when they went into labour, we might be having our babies in supermarkets, or other places that are less than ideal. Labour sensations certainly give us ample warning that we need to snuggle down in our chosen place for birth; in this way, they help us to create that sacred space for ourselves, wherever we have chosen that to be.

Perhaps we become confused by the fact that there is more than one kind of pain; the kind of pain that tells us that something is not right with our body, and the kind of pain that comes from doing hard work for a long time. We "know" that birth is painful because we grow up with this belief so entrenched around us that we cannot possibly help learning this. How different would it feel to grow up in a village where the women experienced joy during their births? Would we approach labour and birth differently if the sensations of labour were called "happies", or "ecstasies" or "joys"? Let's remember that Green's (1991) study showed that women tended to "get what they expected". Here's my idea for a research study: raise fifty young girls without media images of birth, which tend to show women screaming out, and, anytime they ask, tell them that the sensations they will experience during labour and birth are a joyous expression of their womanhood which will take them on a journey more sacred and amazing than they could experience anywhere else. Then see how many of them ask for those sensations to be taken away when they have their babies.

Chapter 14

A Labour of Love

The birth of a child has long been regarded as a rite of passage, an event laden with spiritual meaning, ritual and growth. While the interpretation of this event differs between cultures and philosophies, some generalities exist; the birth of a child not only marks the emergence of a new soul, but the journey of a woman into motherhood, of a man into fatherhood and of the family into a new design which enables continuation of personal and community growth. The circle of life is renewed, and communities rejoice.

Historically, birth traditions and rituals have grown as ways of celebrating and marking this event. As far as we know, women have always gathered together for the birth of a child; older and more experienced women helped those having their first child and were able to draw on their knowledge of physiology, herbs and spiritual rituals to facilitate the process. This is not only a human tendency; several other animals tend to collect together for birth, and dolphins and elephants even have midwives!

We still have birth rituals today, although some of them are vastly different from those our grandmothers would have used. Many of our modern rituals are medical ones; they include inducing labour if it doesn't begin "on time", electronic fetal monitoring, breaking women's waters, using drugs to speed up labour and cutting the cord between mother and baby almost as soon as the baby is born. All of these, as before, can be incredibly useful when used appropriately, and be incredibly harmful, invasive and/or disrespectful of the sacredness of the journey of labour and birth when used routinely.

Most women know that all drugs and interventions carry risks and side effects. As with the example of ultrasound in Chapter 11, the screening tests used during labour and birth, which include fetal monitoring and vaginal examination, can give inaccurate results. False results include both 'false positives', which tend to lead to further unnecessary interventions, and 'false negatives', which lull us into a false sense of security. This is one of my own stories about a 'false negative' result during a woman's labour, which also says a lot about the kinds of knowledge we value:

> *"I was looking after a woman in hospital whose labour had been induced. It was her third baby, and she had a drip containing oxytocin, to get her labour going. Her baby's heartbeat was being monitored, and the tracing coming from the machine looked fine. Yet I felt a bit uncomfortable, worried even, although I couldn't put my finger on why. I had a feeling that the intravenous drugs were not doing this baby any good. A couple of times, I went out to see more senior members of staff, to discuss my concerns with them, and they kept pointing to the fact that the fetal heart monitor showed that the baby's heartbeat was fine and told me not to worry. At one point, the senior doctor said to me, "What do you want me to do ~ a cesarean?! You're normally the one jumping up and down telling me we just need to give the women a bit more time before we do a cesarean!" He was very affable about the whole thing, and he was right ~ I didn't want the women to have a cesarean unnecessarily, but he wasn't prepared to consider the idea that the machine might be wrong."*
>
> *"But I was still worried, and so I made sure I had everything I might need around me if there was a problem, and spent a little time thinking about what would I do if... And I was very glad I did, because, all of a sudden, the baby's heartbeat dropped dramatically, and I had the things I needed around me to deal with it, and I was prepared, almost expecting it. The woman had an emergency cesarean section; the baby was born within seven minutes, and both the woman and her baby were fine. But it was a salutary lesson to me in how the 'false positive' result could actually happen in reality; even if the machine said all was OK right now, that didn't mean everything really was OK. I could so easily have ignored my intuition and been somewhere else (either literally or in my thoughts) just at the moment when I needed to act."*

The other side of this picture is that, as I've mentioned before, some cesareans are carried out unnecessarily because the tracing on the machine suggests there is a problem, where no problem exists in reality. These are the babies who come out screaming $\sim$ I sometimes wonder if they are cross because they have been unnecessarily prevented from finishing their own journey.

Reynolds (1991) talks about the "one-two punch", where one intervention is carried out to solve a problem, and then another intervention is needed to sort out a problem caused by the first intervention. This is also known as "the cascade of intervention" and some examples of this in labour and birth include:

- The artificial rupture of membranes (to break the waters) which is needed because simply being in hospital has slowed down the woman's labour and, rather than suggesting the woman goes home again, staff feel compelled to 'get things going'.
- The opiate drugs (like pethidine) which are needed because the woman experiences so much pain after the artificial rupture of membranes causes her contractions to increase more quickly than if she had remained in natural labour.
- The anti-nausea drugs which are needed to try to reduce the sickness caused by the opiate drugs.
- The intravenous oxytocin drip which is needed because the opiates have again caused labour to slow down or stop.
- The epidural which is needed because the intravenous oxytocin increases the frequency and pain of contractions and causes much more pain than the woman can handle.
- The forceps which are needed because the epidural, which numbs women's muscles, is preventing the woman from feeling the urge to push her baby out.
- The episiotomy, which is needed because the woman's birth canal, which is of more than adequate size to push her baby out, cannot accommodate the extra space needed to get the forceps in.
- The additional drugs needed to get the placenta out, because the drugs given to the woman to speed up her labour have interfered with her own hormones and meant that she would otherwise be in danger of bleeding.

- The artificial milk which is needed because the woman is so exhausted by the whole experience that she doesn't have the energy to persist with breastfeeding.

Interventions often lead to the slowing of labour or interference with the physiological processes which help this work. Episiotomy ~ a cut which is made through the perineum (which is the skin and tissue between the vagina and the anus) and extends the opening of the vagina ~ prevents the rush of the hormone oxytocin which occurs as the baby's head stretches the perineum during birth. The purpose of this rush of oxytocin through a woman's bloodstream is to help the uterus contract and this initiates the birth of the placenta. Cutting the perineum prevents this rush of oxytocin and can lead to unnecessary bleeding. We often seem to forget that women have given birth for many years without the need for routine intervention ~ often, there is a good explanation for why birth works better without it.

Yet, while there is a clear need for women to be informed about the kinds of medical rituals they might be offered, the area which is really neglected is that of the other rituals around birth ~ the social rituals which are personal to us. While these are potentially important for every family, they may become even more important for those women who choose medicalised birth experiences, whether because they have a health issue which makes this the only possible option, or because they do not feel comfortable rejecting the technology on offer.

When anyone becomes a parent, they are taking on a huge responsibility, and they need to feel as strong and confident as possible in order to meet the challenges they will face as a mother or father. Giving responsibility over to someone else and having interventions imposed upon oneself can lead to feelings of dissatisfaction, loss of control and failure. On the other hand, taking responsibility and making choices can help parents to feel strong and well-equipped for their new roles.

For a number of years, women have been encouraged to make "birth plans" ~ which often end up as lists of preferences, stating whether women want to have particular routine interventions or not. Some of these include some of the social aspects of birth, such as whether the baby's father would like to cut the cord, whether the woman would like the baby born onto her tummy, and whether she would like to have skin-to-skin contact with the baby immediately after the birth. But the whole concept of a birth plan assumes that you can "plan" how your labour and birth will happen, and, if you can find a midwife and ask her what she thinks of that idea, you are almost guaranteed a laugh, or at least a kindly speech about how you can't plan something so uncertain.

While we talk about the idea of "taking control" around birth (and I know I have already mentioned this word a few times), birth is something that cannot be controlled. Indeed, women need to give up control and 'go into themselves' in labour in order for the whole journey to happen. It's almost like we have to go to another place in order to make the transition into motherhood. For some women, that place is very sacred. Whatever is happening on the outside, a sacred journey is being undertaken within.

For some women, the answer to the question of whether they will feel able to give up control is to ensure that they will have someone with them in labour who can 'hold a space' around them. That person might be the midwife who is going to attend them or, if they are in a situation where they cannot choose their midwife, a partner, birth companion or doula*. There seems to be something around feeling protected, supported and loved that is a key part of the birth journey for some women.

Several couples I have worked with have also created their own unique rituals for labour and the birth of their baby. Some have gathered special foods to celebrate the onset of labour, and planned music, candle ceremonies or massage oils to use during their birth. Others undertake meditations, or incorporate prayers or mantras into the labour itself, perhaps with the woman choosing a special affirmation or prayer to use during contractions. I know women who have taken "birth boxes" into the hospital, containing lots of things they might like to use. One woman had planned a home birth in a birth pool but finally decided at forty-two weeks of pregnancy that she would have her labour induced in hospital. She held a "birth party", both to celebrate the dawn of her labour and to get used to the idea that she was giving up her home birth. The night before she went to the hospital, she dimmed the lights, got into the birth pool with her partner, and 'went inside' to connect with her baby. This, she said later, was vitally important to her journey, and enabled her to let go of her hopes of birthing

---

* "Doula" is the term used for a professional or personal birth attendant. The word itself is Greek and translates as 'woman's servant'.

this baby at home. (Her second baby was born at home, and came so quickly that the midwife made it with only minutes to spare. That time, the pool was refilled the next day and the whole family held the birth party to celebrate their new baby being twenty-four hours old.)

One woman who did not have a partner felt that she wished to connect with the other women in her life. She invited them to a special party a few weeks before her birth, and bring something which she could use to connect with the energy of birth, while stressing that she was not asking for expensive presents. Some of her friends brought stones, crystals or dried flowers, while others brought items which they had found useful in their own births; lavender massage oil, herbal tea, aromatherapy candles and a pair of woolly socks! (Many women find that, although they do not want the restriction of clothes, their feet get cold during labour.) Through these gifts, and her own work, she felt empowered and surrounded by love and energy during her birth, which was also attended by three of these women.

Of course, birth rituals do not have to be based on material items alone. Because of the link between the moon, tides and women's cycles, some women like to visit the sea in the days or weeks leading up to their births. One woman spent her pregnancy planning and tending a herb garden, which she then spent most of her labour in. She read up on the herbs which were the most beneficial to labour, and grew these together in an arbor which later also became the site for an apple tree planted over the baby's placenta. I attended a home birth once where the older children collected some of the air from the birth in jam jars ~ they both sensed that this was a special and spiritual event, and wanted a keepsake to help them recapture this feeling.

Birth rituals can benefit women, babies and their families. When we understand that the newly born baby is a unique and fully-grown soul who just happens to be in a little body and welcome babies with gentle actions and kind words, perhaps it matters less where and how they are born. I have seen several babies who arrive in the world disorientated, yet who soon recover when we explain that they are at the end of their journey and are with those who love them. Likewise, when we understand that birth is an incredible rite of passage of women and those around them, we can find ways which help us make meaning of this experience for ourselves. Whatever other choices we make, and whatever other choices are made for us, we always have the choice to experience labour and birth as a sacred journey.

Chapter 15

A Sourcebook of Pregnancy and Birth Choices

In Chapter 10, I talked about the wise woman tradition, and the different steps of healing outlined by Weed (1989). These steps are incredibly useful as a tool to think about the options when you are experiencing an issue or problem which you would like to address or heal. They can equally be used when pregnant or birthing women and new mothers experience a problem; there are often many things that can be tried, which would come in the first few steps, before resorting to pharmaceutical supplements, drugs or surgery. Supplements, drugs and surgery can, of course, be very useful, and sometimes life-saving, but there is little doubt that we over-use them, creating potential problems for ourselves and our children. Some of the non-medical options are not yet well known and understood by pregnant women, and, perhaps because of the dominance of the medical model during the past few decades, some of these are only now being written down and debated*.

However, while some pregnant women will experience problems that they need to think through, almost all pregnant women will be offered a variety of tests and interventions for themselves and their babies, and this is another area where tools to think about the options can be very useful. A few years ago, I developed a way of categorising interventions into four main categories, which, although is only one way of looking at such issues, have helped some women think through the issues relating to the things that they are being offered (Wickham 2002). These categories are:

1. Screening tests
2. Clinical interventions

---

* Some web-based sources of this kind of knowledge can be found in the links on www.withwoman.co.uk

3. Prophylactic interventions
4. Selected interventions.

Each of these types of intervention is offered for a slightly different reason. Because of this, there are specific questions which can be asked about each which will help you gain the information you need to help you make decisions about whether or not you and your baby will benefit from them. The sections below outline the reasoning behind each type of intervention and the kinds of questions you could ask when gathering information about them from your birth attendant and other sources. These tools, by the way, are not limited to interventions around childbirth; this model can equally be applied in other areas of health and it is complementary to other tools, such as the "six steps of healing".

Screening tests

Screening tests are designed to detect 'deviations from the normal'. These tests may be carried out to detect deviations from the normal in the woman or the baby (or babies). Sometimes the interventions are carried out on the woman, but are actually screening the baby. An example of this is where a midwife palpates, or feels, the woman's abdomen during pregnancy; among other things, she is determining whether the baby is growing within normal limits or whether the growth of the baby has 'deviated from the normal'. Although many screening tests have been challenged within the lay and professional literature, most are still a feature of routine practice, yet women are fully entitled to decline them and still receive respectful treatment.

Examples of screening tests include ultrasound, vaginal examination, fetal blood sampling, antenatal 'checks', blood tests, postnatal (after the birth) checks and blood pressure testing. If you think about it, all of these things are done to see whether you and your body (and perhaps baby) are 'normal', or whether you have a deviation from the norm, which might be perceived as a problem.

The benefit of a screening test lies in the accuracy with which we can define 'normal'. While in some areas there is a generally accepted range of what 'normal' is, in others there is disagreement. The other important question to ask yourself (or your midwife) is whether, if some aspect of your or your baby's health is found to be 'outside normal limits' in some way, can anything be done about this? For instance, if you have high blood pressure, there are treatments which can reduce this which you can consider taking. On the other hand, if your baby is found to be growing more slowly than normal, as was the case for Emma in Chapter 11, there is very little that can be done to change this. The information that there may be a deviation from the norm can, however, lead to unnecessary worry.

Some important questions to ask of any screening test that you are offered include:

- How accurate is the test? (Some have a wide margin for error).
- What are the risks of getting a false result? (This includes being told that all is well when actually it is not, and being told that there is a problem when this is not the case.)
- What will the psychological impact of the test be? (Many women find that waiting for the results of tests, particularly for antenatal screening, is very stressful. You may want to talk through how you would cope with your partner or family or friends before agreeing to the test.)
- How are 'normal limits' defined in this area? (Is there general agreement on this? Do you agree with the attendant's definition of normal?)
- Is the outcome of the screening test going to affect the choices I can make?
- If the outcome shows a deviation from the norm, is there anything that can be done about this? (Ask yourself also if the answer to this question is something which you would accept. For instance, if you consented to a vaginal examination and were told that you had ~ in the attendant's opinion ~ not made satisfactory progress, would you want to have your labour speeded up or, assuming that all was otherwise well with both you and your baby, would you prefer to continue labouring at your own pace?)

Clinical interventions

Usually used following a screening test, clinical interventions are used to bring pregnancy/labour/the situation back in line with 'normal limits'. In the example above, acceleration of labour would be the clinical intervention that might follow the use of vaginal examination as a screening test to determine whether labour was progressing at 'normal speed'. Clinical interventions should be used on an individual basis ～ in response to the needs of an individual woman rather than as a routine part of care. However, some attendants still use some clinical interventions routinely, for instance by inducing all women's labours at a certain stage of pregnancy.

Examples of clinical interventions include induction of labour, blood transfusion, breaking your waters, speeding up labour, forceps or vacuum delivery and emergency cesarean section. In contrast to the "six steps of healing" model, where you might consider different levels of intervention if you suspected a problem, the interventions offered usually come into the later categories, of drugs and surgical intervention. That does not mean, of course, that you couldn't take the information gained in a screening test and think about whether you wanted to try other things in the "six steps" model before you resorted to drugs or surgery.

This is another area where the question of 'what is normal' arises ～ do your ideas of normality agree with those of your attendant or the institution you are giving birth in? How accurate was the screening test on which the suggestion for this intervention was based? Decisions need to be based on an understanding of what is likely happen if things are left to continue versus what is likely to happen if you consent to intervention. The word "BRAN" can be helpful in this situation, where you ask:

What are the **B**enefits?
What are the **R**isks?
What are the **A**lternatives?
What happens if I do **N**othing?

Other questions to think about if you are offered a clinical intervention include:

- What is the range of possibilities if I agree to this intervention, and how likely is each of these?
- What is the range of possibilities if I do not agree to this intervention, and how likely is each of these?
- Does the intervention usually work? For what proportion of women/babies?
- What are the physical, psychological and other risks of this intervention?

- What are the side effects of this intervention? (How do you feel about these? Are they greater or lesser than the possible outcomes if you choose to wait a while and reassess the situation?)
- Is there a possibility that this intervention will lead to a 'cascade of intervention'? (As discussed in Chapter 14). How do I feel about this possibility?

Prophylactic interventions

Prophylactic interventions are used 'just in case' to prevent potential problems from occurring. Usually the problem that they aim to prevent will only happen occasionally, but the intervention will be offered to many women and/or babies in the hope that the few who would have experienced the problem are among those who have taken up prophylactic treatment. Prophylactic interventions do not themselves give information on the likelihood of a problem occurring, nor are they used ~ on the whole ~ with screening or other tests which could give information on this.

Examples of prophylactic interventions include antenatal anti-D for rhesus negative women, vitamin K for newborn babies, antibiotics for women in preterm labour, or where they are thought to be at risk from infections such as Group B strep, withholding food and fluids from women in labour and induction of labour once a certain point of pregnancy has been reached.

There are a number of philosophical issues that relate to the use of prophylactic interventions. Is it appropriate to give these to all women or babies when only a few will benefit? Are there other ways of establishing whether a particular woman or baby is at risk? Are the side effects of prophylactic interventions justified for all of the women and babies who turn out not to have been at risk? For instance, if women are prevented from eating and drinking in labour because this may be of benefit if they end up having a cesarean section (although this itself is debatable), they may then be more likely to need other interventions in their labour as they become hungry, thirsty, tired and in need of the energy that would have been provided if they had been able to eat and drink. Do the possible benefits to the few women who need an emergency cesarean section outweigh the risks of increased intervention to all women who accept this kind of prophylaxis?

Questions to think about before you accept a prophylactic intervention include:

- What percentage of people actually end up in the situation that this intervention is designed to prevent? Am I likely to be one of those women? (Or, is my baby likely to be one of those babies?)
- If I ~ or my baby or babies ~ ends up in that situation, what can be done to deal with it then?
- Does the prophylactic intervention actually work? In how many cases does it do what it is meant to do? How often does it fail?
- What are the risks of the prophylactic intervention to me and/or my baby?
- Do I believe that the potential benefits of the prophylactic intervention outweigh the risks?

Selected interventions

Finally, selected interventions are those interventions which may or may not be related to the health or progress of pregnancy, birth or the postpartum/neonatal period, but which are still used by a proportion of women. They may be deliberately requested and chosen by women themselves, or women may be advised to consider them by attendants.

Examples of selected interventions include pain relief (which may be non-pharmacological, e.g. TENS, massage, herbs or pharmacological, e.g. epidural, narcotics, entonox), elective cesarean section (where the woman has requested this) and using water for labour and birth.

One of the most significant questions in relation to a selected intervention is whether the woman herself wants this intervention ~ and why. Interestingly, this category not only includes some of the most potentially dangerous interventions in childbirth ~ such as epidural and cesarean section ~ but also some of those which women have been choosing since time immemorial, such as using warm water and massage to relieve pain in labour. The question of whether some of these interventions, especially elective cesarean section, should be an option for all women is an emotive issue which raises interesting ethical issues in relation to choice.

Questions to ask around selected interventions include:

- Do I feel the use of this intervention will be of benefit to me, my baby and/or my labour and birth experience?
- What are the benefits and risks of this intervention?
- Do the benefits of this intervention outweigh the risks of it for me as an individual?
- If I decide I want this intervention or therapy, am I able to achieve this locally, or do I need to think about going further afield or talking to other people who might be able to help me?

As I have spent much of this chapter dealing with some of the issues surrounding the more medical aspects of pregnancy and birth, and raising questions about some of the aspects of the pregnancy and birth journey which some women may want to avoid, I wanted to finish with a list of positive things that women have told me they have done for themselves or another woman during pregnancy and birth, which would come in the "engage the energy" step...

- During pregnancy, invite each of your women friends to give you a bead or trinket, which you can then make into a bracelet or necklace to wear during labour...
- Focus on visualising your body allowing your baby to be born simply, easily, happily and in love...
- Find out about the birth traditions which exist in your part of the world, to see if you would like to include any of these in your plans...
- Invite the women who are close to you to join you for an evening and share positive experiences and advice with you...
- Ensure that, if you are reading books on pregnancy, birth and the early postnatal/mothering period, they are both positive and aligned with your own feelings about the experience.
- Consider keeping a journal or diary of your pregnancy, perhaps for you, or for you and your partner, or to give to your baby when she or he is old enough to understand...
- Investigate some of the traditional and modern rituals around the placenta, so you can either think about whether you would like to honour

your baby's placenta in some way, or else marvel at the things other women do...

- Think beyond the birth about what you might need, and ask your friends and family if they might be able to help and provide some of these things so that you know you will have support if and when you need it ∼ this can be material things for you and the baby, practical help, or emotional or spiritual support...

- Find out how to make a dreamcatcher for your baby, and choose the thread, beads and feathers while thinking about what you would like for your baby (remembering, of course, that she or he will surprise you in almost every way possible!)

Chapter 16

The Mother–Baby Spiral

Les cerfs-volants	**Kites**
Je t'ai vue	I saw you
la tête inclinée	your head tilted
ton chapeau de paille	your straw hat
attaché à ton doux menton	tied to your soft chin
par un ruban de toutes les couleurs	with a ribbon of all colours
tes mains empoignant de toute	your hands, holding with all
leur force	their might
le long fil	the long thread
qui te reliait	which linked you
à ton cerf-volant	to your kite
dans tes yeux, que je ne	in your eyes, which I could
pouvais voir	not see
le vent avait ouvert	the wind had opened
un grand horizon	a wide horizon
où volaient tous les cerf-volants	where all the kites of childhood
de l'enfance	were flying
grands carrés multicolores	great multicoloured squares
flottant dans la mare	floating in the dark and
sombre et profonde	deep pond
de ton regard	of your gaze
envoûté	spell-bound
je t'ai vue	I saw you
la tête à peine émergée	your head just emerged
de la chaleur de mon corps	from the heat of my body
le long fil	the long thread

qui te reliait	which linked you
au cœur de mon ventre	to the heart of my womb
encore vibrant	still vibrant
tes yeux noirs	your black eyes
avides de découvrir le monde	eager to discover the world
dans mes yeux	in my eyes
les milliers de cerf-volants	the thousand of kites
que tu allais faire voler	which you would fly one day

Sophie Bérubé (2002)

If you ask an eighty-year-old British woman what she did in the first few days after her babies were born, she will probably tell you about "lying-in", where she and her baby would stay in bed together for a couple of weeks after the birth and be excused from doing any work. If you ask a British woman in her fifties, she might tell you that lying-in was thought to be a bit old-fashioned by the time she had babies; several of the women of this generation who I talked to said they stayed in bed for a couple of days after their babies were born, but then pretty much *"got up and got on with it"*. Yet, ask a woman who is currently pregnant, especially one who knows a lot about different birth options, and she just might tell you about the 'babymoon' ~ an apparently new idea which, if we look at it more closely, is really a re-vision of a fairly ancient one.

This is, by the way, by no means an idea unique to Britain, and it is certainly not a Western creation. Many Native American Indian tribes have a variation of this, as do cultures which originated in India, South America and Africa, although the length of time which mother and baby spend in seclusion varies between cultures. The term 'babymoon' was coined by Sheila Kitzinger, an anthropologist who has written extensively about birth. It plays on the word 'honeymoon': a time where a couple take space to be together and enjoy each other following their marriage. Taking a few days weeks away from normal life and chores can help with recovery from a hectic and possibly stressful few weeks and it can provide space to foster new family relationships and make the transition into parenthood.

Ancient ideas such as this one often seem to spiral around to become modern ones, although sometimes with additions, and this is no exception. Like menstrual seclusion, the idea that a woman needs to be secluded after childbirth because she is 'dirty' has been interpreted in some circles as a negative and anti-feminist belief, where in reality the story may simply have become jumbled in the telling. But this is not to say that the ancient and modern babymoons are entirely similar. Where lying-in was generally about a mother and her baby, the babymoon often includes the woman's partner and any other children they have as well. Unlike the lying-in period, signs politely asking prospective visitors to give the new family some space often accompany the modern babymoon, and couples sometimes use the technology of e-mail to send out news and photos of the new baby in an attempt to placate relatives desperate to see the new arrival. While help in the form of housework or food preparation is welcomed, intrusion is not, and some couples choose to ask a close relative or friend to help protect their space by acting as an interface between them and the outside world:

> *"We got my mum to let people know we had had the baby, but that we didn't want to be disturbed. And we put a sign on the gate with a picture of the baby saying she was here and we were enjoying our time as a family but we would bring her out when we all felt ready. I'm sure some people thought it wasn't OK, but we made the decision not to care. Some people dropped off food, though, they would just knock and leave something on the doorstep. That was so great."*
>
> (Marguerite)

> *"It was a really precious time. I wish I had done it with my first baby, I'll definitely do it again if we have another."*
>
> (Claire)

In some cultures, women and their families also celebrate the day their baby is nine months old. It is seen as a significant day because that is the day that the baby becomes seen as a separate person; until then, baby and mother are one. This, like the babymoon, furthers the idea that mother and baby remain as one for long after the birth, and that the process of separation is gradual rather than abrupt. Yet this is in stark contrast to some of the modern medical rituals which have been practised immediately after birth and during the early postnatal period over the last few decades, including the practice of taking babies away to a separate nursery and the idea of cutting the baby's cord soon after birth. Although most women do not have their babies taken away to another room nowadays, there is still, in some areas, a focus on cutting the cord fairly soon after birth (a 'privilege' which midwives are now quite likely to offer to the woman's partner) and on having a professional 'check' and dress the baby quickly, sometimes before the woman has had the chance to really look at the baby herself. All of this may further underline the idea that mother and baby are separate beings.

It is difficult to know whether lotus birth ~ the practice of leaving the baby attached to her whole placenta until it falls off naturally a few days after birth ~ is an ancient idea, but it is certainly another which has a small but growing following in modern times. Many believe that this allows a more gentle transition for the baby, and enables the child to have an element of choice in when she leaves her 'tree of life' behind and becomes truly independent in the world. We do know that the last few generations of people in the West have generally discarded and disregarded the placenta, its only real value being economic, and then only during the days before increased knowledge about blood-borne infection, when some hospital sold women's placentas (generally without their knowledge) to cosmetic companies where they were processed to make ingredients for expensive face creams.

Yet some cultures have long regarded the placenta as a sacred organ belonging to the baby, while others esteem the nutritional or medicinal value of the placenta to the new mother. Whether women are choosing to bury, eat or dry their placenta, or leave it attached to their babies until it falls off naturally, there is a noticeable increase in the way we are becoming more conscious of this incredible organ. Unfortunately, as I mentioned above, we cannot say for sure whether lotus birth is an entirely new ritual, or one which is ancient; to my knowledge, no one has found any evidence that it was practised in the distant past. Equally, no one has found any evidence that it was not and, as Michel Odent points out in his introduction to "Lotus Birth", we need to re-learn what birth can be like when it is not disturbed, using non-interventive reference points such as lotus birth in order to do so.

Two aspects of lotus birth have always struck me as especially interesting. One is the marked difference which having the placenta still attached (albeit usually contained in a bag or parcel) makes to the degree to which the baby can be passed around to relatives and friends. If a family do not have a babymoon, and other people are around them, lotus birth makes it far more difficult to play the kind of "pass-the-parcel" game that is often a feature of a baby's first few days on Earth.

The other is the question of whether the placenta 'belongs' to the mother or her baby, which then raises the equally important question of whether it is fair to cut the cord before the baby is 'ready' to release the placenta, or fair for the mother to eat the placenta. On a pragmatic level we might decide that, as parents, we have to make all kinds of choices for our children before they become ready to do so themselves, and this is simply one more that we simply have to make for them to the best of our ability. On the other hand, some of the midwives who have started to use the term motherbaby to reinforce their assertion that the woman and baby remain one (or two-in-one) for some time after birth as well as during pregnancy would probably argue that, as the two cannot easily be separated, the placenta belongs to both.

If we put together the rituals of lotus birth, of the babymoon and of seeing motherbaby as one until nine months have passed, the one thing that links them is the idea of connection ~ a far longer, more passionate and firmer connection than we currently honour in our society. It has been more than two decades since Starhawk (1982) pointed out that we need to focus more on connections; that if we continue to believe in separation, of body and mind, of matter and spirit, of concepts, of people, of decisions, of mother and baby, we will continue to live in a world of estrangement. Perhaps the re-emergence of some of these old ideas, albeit in a new form, might mean that we are beginning to take these ideas on board. I can't think of any better place for such ideas to grow than in the (connected) hearts and minds of the women who will teach the next generation.

Chapter 17

Mothers and Mothering

Le réveil	awakening
je connais ton sommeil	I know your slumber
comme la niche de mon ventre	like the nook of my belly
dans un pacte de flanalette	in a pact of flannelette
de duvet et d'orteils réchauffés	of dawn and warmed-up toes
tes yeux encore un peu incrustés d'étoiles	your eyes still slightly incrusted with stars
je peux respirer	I can breathe
sur ta petite bouche	on your little mouth
la sensation de rêves	the sensation of dreams
que j'ai déjà portés	that I have already carried

Sophie Bérubé (2002)

Mothers are all around us: our own and other people's ~ in our own lives, in the street, and on our TV screens. They come in all shapes, sizes and types, from the well-attended glamorous celebrity mother leaving the private hospital after her scheduled cesarean to the harried mother trying to cope in a busy supermarket with a limited budget and two screaming toddlers who don't understand why they can't have the colourful sweeties, so carefully placed by the marketing experts to be in such easy reach of their fingers. As modern role models, we can choose from the super-slim and in-control (despite having apparently recently given birth) mothers who advertise baby products, the washing-powder mothers who have nothing more to do with their days than invite male celebrities in to watch them wash their son's football strips, or the cordon-bleu mothers who feed their children a range of foods of varying nutritional levels while always retaining a sense of humour in the face of adversity. If somebody would only use the barely-coping-and-trying-not-to-yell-at-the-kids-but-not-quite-making-it model of mother to advertise a product, I'd be tempted go straight out and buy whatever they were selling. There is, for many women, a substantial and striking difference between the images of mothering that see in the media, and the reality of this spiral.

I asked mothers, both during interviews and via e-mail, what advice that they would give to a woman who was becoming a mother for the first time. The fact that so many of them mentioned the need for women to understand that they could not live up to the images and expectations our society has of mothers suggests to me that this is a serious issue for modern women. It is often said that to be a mother is the hardest job imaginable, and, while it may well also be the most rewarding, there is no limit to the people who feel they are entitled to voice opinions about the way that individual women choose to carry out this role.

Other advice that mothers would offer to women who were becoming mothers included the understanding that there will be plenty of advice on offer, and some of it is very useful, but that mothers need to figure out what works for them as individuals:

> *"To go with her body ... to love her body ... to find a midwife who is 'with woman' and to ask as many questions as she wants"*
>
> (Rachel)

> *"My first thought was ... don't do it! Sorry ... only joking! But having a son [of] sixteen who knows it all better and a daughter now thirteen, its difficult to remember what it was first like. Listen to other young mums and take the advice you think sounds right. My sister has now got a seven-month-old daughter and when I am with her I'm so much more relaxed than she is. It's her second one. You learn through the mistakes you are making but become a better mum. Nobody was born to be a mother and I followed that thought ... so you only learn through the mistakes and pass the good and bad thoughts on to others."*
>
> (Kath)

"Take each day at a time and don't punish yourself ... some days you'll feel great. At others exhausted, so pace yourself ... and don't fret if your key result areas don't get completed ~ they will tomorrow, or the day after! In the first year you may think you will never be able to get out again ~ it isn't true. By the time they are teenagers they will be the one who is out all the time and you'll just want to go to bed!!"

(Rebecca)

"The one thing I do remember is a little old nun at the hospital saying 'once you are home, listen to all the good advice from friends and relations, be polite to them and thank them ... and then do your own thing!'"

(Lise)

"I would say, do what you feel is best for you and your child and ask questions about whatever you are in doubt about."

(Joan)

"Advice is just that, ADVICE, take of it what you want, there is no right or wrong way ... you just do what you've got to do to get through, you will learn as you go. It's like a baptism of fire and even if you think you're prepared you won't be ... It's a very steep learning curve and you WILL get through it. All the thoughts that you had on how it would be and how you would feel go out of the window and I personally really appreciated my mum when I became one!!"

(Lou)

"My first reaction is to suggest 'don't listen to any advice'! That sounds a bit facile, but I think pregnant women, those who have recently given birth and those who are vocalising their wish to be pregnant get bombarded with advice, suggestions and comments. A lot of it may be well meaning but a lot of it is also nonsense, alarming and unhelpful. So, I suppose my comment would be to point out to women that this will happen, and to suggest that they learn to smile politely but choose to ignore *as much of it as they want. I would suggest that they will know instinctively what is best for their baby, who will be a completely unique individual and quite unlike any other baby that has been, or will be born and therefore they can relax and trust their own judgement. And then I would want them to enjoy being pregnant ... being a mother ... planning the pregnancy because it is a precious time. So I suppose my three guiding principles are trust your instincts, relax and enjoy it!"*

(Monica)

It was interesting that the advice to trust one's instincts and enjoy the experience of being a mother came up several times...

"Trust your instinct and enjoy ... oh yes ... and remember to giggle"

(Alice)

"Try and be instinctive ~ whilst listening to 'everyone', please yourself in terms of mothering style etc. Of course the most important one to listen to is your child ~ including non verbal cues. And enjoy!"

(Genevieve)

Some women offered practical advice too:

"I also really like the advice that one of my friends who is a midwife and health visitor and midwife and had her three children very close together, gave to my sister in law. 'Really' she said, 'the only thing you need to know is that mashed banana never washes out of the baby clothes'!"

(Monica)

"Pear is difficult too."

(Alice)

"Don't expect to be a perfect mother: there's no such thing! Children need breathing space as much as mums do ~ don't over-look the willing support systems provided by grandparents ~ they

don't want to take over, believe me ... they will be only too happy to hand back at the end of the day! Green peppers, raisins and ice cream make a balanced diet ... [this is] not a product of my own imagination ... and baked beans on toast is full of fibre and nutrition. And adults do know best most of the time ... autonomy for small children leads to insecurity and a small tyrant. [That's] not PC, I know... Good parenting is not an exercise in popularity. And above all ... Babies are tough!"

(Marilyn)

"Communicate, communicate, communicate ~ having a new one in your life changes everything and you need to make sure you try and share the load with your partner and the people who are around you. Recognise that all your relationships will change ~ you may feel different towards friends who have no children, your parents may find being a grandparent tough or great, your partner may find the changes in you and your life difficult ~ so communicate, communicate, communicate again! And don't be too proud to ask for help ~ or to accept help that is offered ~ you can reciprocate later when you are less busy."

(Rebecca)

Marilyn also had advice for adoptive mothers:

"You will never measure up to the 'perfect' birth mother as you have to cope with day to day reality. It's not a fair competition. However, be assured you have your own place that is unique."

(Marilyn)

And a midwife friend e-mailed this to me the day after she had run a 'parentcraft' session for couples expecting their first baby:

"I do often finish off ante natal classes with a little word like this actually... Sometimes it goes down well and sometimes it falls completely flat (like last night). It is a test of us as parents how we cope with our children's failures/disappointments/

shortcomings. This of course is not a problem straightaway but will become apparent with the rush of years and we have to hold on to what we have and not be over impressed by secondary concerns ~ e.g. good at sports/school, slim, witty, sparkling personality, whatever our hearts hold dear to us in our little anal worlds, we have to say; Get a life, it just doesn't matter!"

(Harriet)

While I was researching for this book, I gave the women who let me interview them an information sheet about the project, and asked them to fill out a form with a few details about themselves. One of the questions on the form was simply "number of children". As I went through the pile of forms one day, to check I had everybody's code-name correct, I noticed that very few women had left this question blank. As you might expect, those women who have children had written in the number of children they had, and sometimes their names and ages. Several women had also written about children they had conceived but who, for whatever reason, had never seen life on this planet, and children they had taken care of when other mothers needed help. A few women didn't list human children but detailed cats, dogs and rabbits, and a couple of women used this space to write about non-human 'babies'. These included projects they had managed (or perhaps that should be womanaged), books they had written and things they had achieved in their life.

While there is a real need to honour mothers in our society, there is also a need to honour women who aren't mothers, or who are mothers in other ways. In *The Blue Jay's Dance*, Erdrich (1995) suggests that women without children can be the best of mothers, perhaps because they carry more patience, interest and clarity of focus than can be sustained by those who are constantly with their children. SARK agrees that women have a maternal gift, a divine ability to nurture, commenting that:

"We are all mothers in special ways. Godmothers, big sisters, aunts, or simply friends with children. There are so many children already here who need love ~ it isn't necessary to be a mother to experience mothering."

(SARK 1997: 99)

I went back to a few women, some of whom were mothers, some of whom were midwives and some of whom were neither, and asked for their thoughts on this:

"In society's eyes I am not a mother as I do not have any biological children ... I do feel there is an odd attitude to 'traditional' motherhood in our society as, on one level it is greatly honoured and valued and I feel as though I am seen as an oddity because I do not have my own children. I get very tired of questions such as 'do you have a family?' which is a ridiculous question because of course everyone has some sort of family, however dysfunctional or perfect. What they mean is 'do you have children?' I find it particularly grating as a midwife when asked if I have children as I feel that some sort of value judgement is made about me when I say 'no'. The last few times it happened I replied, 'no, it didn't happen for me', which seemed to end the inquisition! I suppose what I would like to say to the question 'do you have children' is 'no, but does that matter to you, because I am OK with that reality? I feel I am as 'worthwhile' and womanly as any woman who has had her own biological children."

(Melissa)

"I believe that all women are capable of 'mothering', as you say both children and 'projects' etc. However, many women hold back, or choose not to be open to this side of their nature. I think that if they could recognise this, their lives would be enhanced by opening up to this part of themselves. In fact, I think it is part of the root of so many problems worldwide. That is, the world, its' people and places are so often no longer 'mothered', as women spend so much time and energy on themselves ~ the opposite of a woman's purpose, perhaps ~ that of the 'giver'. Men, have always been 'takers' ~ sadly many women are also now 'takers'."

(Genevieve)

"I'm not a mother, I would like to have been, but it wasn't meant to be. In some ways I have been a mother my whole life,

maybe now I need to stop ... It's hard to know where to put my mothering energy though ..."

(Debbie)

"I feel motherly a lot! I think midwives are motherly. I feel responsible, caring and supportive and I sometimes loose sleep worrying about cases etc ... isn't that a motherly instinct? Don't you think women have a motherly essence about them? Well perhaps not all women but I certainly have motherly feelings to inanimate objects, animals, friends, even people I see on the telly!! Maybe I've lost the plot!"

(Lou)

I don't think Lou has lost the plot at all; for what my opinion is worth, she is one of the most down-to-earth women I have ever met. When you compare the complex reality of these women's words to the rose-tinted images and depictions of mothers and children, it might seem ever more important to work on ways in which we can enable women to learn from and honour each other's experiences; taking what works for them, rejecting what doesn't, and holding a space where all kinds of mothering are valued as personal, 'good enough' and sacred.

Chapter 18

Sacred Milk

In Greek mythology, the God Zeus, who was married to the Goddess Hera, had a child with a mortal woman, Alcmene. Although you may not have heard of Alcmene, you may well have heard of her child, Hercules. Zeus, like any good parent, wanted Hercules to be immortal, but, unlike most parents, he knew how to achieve this; by giving Hercules a taste of the immortality in the sacred fluid of Hera's milk. So Zeus sneaked Hercules into Hera's bedroom and put him to her breast while she was sleeping. However, Hercules' vigorous suckling woke Hera up and, displeased at what Zeus had done, she shook Hercules off her breast. Because breast milk often continues to flow, and because Hera was moving to remove Hercules from her breast, her milk spurted across the sky, forming the Milky Way.

Sometime between Ancient Greece and modern times, breast milk has lost its status as a life-giving, sacred fluid. It might not have become quite as vilified as menstrual blood, but society has variously attempted to hide it away in public toilets (which are places I would never want to eat my lunch), remove it from view in restaurants and even, thanks to a woman Speaker, ban it in House of Commons' committees (Palmer 2003). Breast milk has suffered further insult from the big business of artificial milks, which erroneously claim their products are almost as good, and, as awareness of environmental issues increases, from claims that it is polluted. (As Steingraber (2001) suggests, it is the world that is polluted and about which we really ought to be worried, not breast milk, which is merely a reflection of the level of pollution of the Earth herself). When you add the denigration of breast milk to society's changing perception of breasts and the half-truths which women have been fed about breastfeeding, it is little wonder that only about a quarter of three-month-old babies are still enjoying their mother's milk.

About ten years ago, I was in a shopping mall somewhere in Michigan with a friend of mine who had a six-month-old baby. Her baby needed to feed, and we sat down together on a bench where she quietly breastfed. Several people glanced at us, but no one said anything until a woman walked by, did a double take and then made a loud tutting sound, saying something that we didn't catch but which sounded disapproving. She walked a few more steps and then turned around. I felt my own maternal instincts rise as I prepared to verbally defend my friend and her child, but instead the woman's face softened. "I shouldn't have done that", she said. "I'm sorry. I'm actually really proud of you." She then smiled, turned and walked away.

I've never really been able to work out what went on for that woman in the few steps between when she first reacted to the sight of my friend breastfeeding and when she turned around and apologised. I wonder if she realised, in those moments, that the reaction she had first displayed was not what she felt, but what she perceived society expected of her. Perhaps it then took another moment for her to realise how it was that she truly felt about the situation, and to this day I honour her courage and humility for turning around and apologising.

There is an acute need to address the lies and manipulations which we have been fed about breasts, breast milk and breastfeeding, but without forcing women to make the decision to breastfeed if this is truly not for them. Some women are simply not comfortable with the idea and, given the decades of poor press which breastfeeding has experienced and the fact that women (especially those who are mothers) have enough other things which they have been trained to feel guilty about, there is no justification for attempting to make women feel bad about the choices they are making.

In many ways, we should celebrate the fact that women who live in the West have the option to artificially feed their babies; thanks to the widespread availability of good sanitation, clean water supplies and treatments for babies who do get sick without their mother's antibodies, it is not an unreasonable choice to make. Women who choose to artificially feed their babies often know that cows' milk formula it is not as good as their own milk; the 'breast is best' campaigns have been around long enough to have had the desired impact, and, often, it is practical, personal and social factors which force their choice. In the words of Angier:

> *"Can we not forgo the polemics and exercise a little more maternal compassion here? In the real world of the two-career family, most women will breastfeed for the first few weeks or months... Like women throughout history they will do the best they can under the constraints of work, duty, and desire. They will be generous and selfish, mammals and magicians, and they will flow and stop flowing. Whatever they do they will feel guilty for not doing enough, and they will wish that they too could drink from the breast of Mary or Hera, thus becoming immortal mothers whose children will never die."*
>
> (Angier 1999: 160–1)

In looking at how we could reclaim a sacred space for breast milk and breastfeeding, Midwife Ina May Gaskin (2003) has diagnosed our society as suffering from a disease she calls 'nipplephobia'. She sees the situation where women do not feel comfortable breastfeeding in public as symptomatic of a social epidemic, and suggests the cure for this would be for our society to be exposed to breasts and breastfeeding on a large scale. Certainly the veneration of breasts as sexual objects has not helped the cause of breastfeeding as a sacred pursuit, and the issue of sexuality and breastfeeding has become very muddled.

Breastfeeding, as well as being a sacred connection between mother and baby, happens to feel very good. It feels good in a similar way to the way that a woman feels good when a lover caresses and suckles at her breasts. That is not to say that some women don't experience some discomfort, even occasional pain, as they learn the ancient skill of breastfeeding which is still new to them, but this is usually fleeting compared to the physical and emotional rewards that breastfeeding can bring. During a feed, oxytocin ~ the hormone which Odent (2001) describes as the 'hormone of love' ~ is released. Because oxytocin is also released during lovemaking, and at birth, there are parallels between these experiences, all of which could be described as sensual. It is, arguably, our attempts to sanitise and clinicise the natural experiences of birth and breastfeeding, perhaps for the benefit of the professionals involved, which have led to our forgetting that these are sensual experiences. Concurrently, we have seen the development of confusion among women about what their breasts are for, which has certainly not been helped by the utilisation of women' breasts in advertising and newspaper sales. Sadly, as Davina's comments in Chapter 6 illustrated, many women today grow up to be ashamed of their breasts, rather than proud of them.

I find breasts and breast milk and breastfeeding amazing. Through our milk, and the maze of tissues, pools, streams and outlets that make, store and dispense it, our breasts are infinitely capable of sustaining the needs of bodies of our children. I have known a woman to happily and success- fully breastfeed triplets until they were a year old, and several women who have simultaneously breastfed two children born a year or two apart. I have met grandmothers who, having weaned their own children two or three decades before, breastfed their grandchildren when their own mothers couldn't, proving that their ability to lactate doesn't stop at menopause, and I know of young girls and women who have never been pregnant who spontaneously create breast milk when they hear a baby cry.

Breastfeeding protects women as well as babies. Palmer (2003) lists research showing that women who have breastfed have lower rates of breast, ovarian and endometrial cancers, and that, under certain circum- stances, fully breastfeeding women are protected from becoming preg- nant again more quickly than their body could handle. She finds it amazing that so many women are more likely to view breasts in terms of their vulnerability, such as in relation to the risk of breasts becoming cancerous, rather than in terms of their power:

> "Breastfeeding has been perceived as a symbol of women's domestication and oppression, but it is an act of power and strength."
>
> (Palmer 2003: 100)

As an act of strength, which is unique to women and associated with blood ~ for breast milk can be described as a blood product, rich as it is in the antibodies and immune protection factors which course through our own blood ~ breastfeeding, like menstruation, birth and menopause, could be described as a blood rite. Curiously, although elsewhere in these pages you'll find examples of celebrations of the other blood rites, the rites where the blood comes from the vagina, I've never heard of anyone celebrating the blood rite of breastfeeding. There are certainly support groups for women who breastfeed, which fulfil the need some women have for sharing of information and experiences, and in some ways these could be seen as a celebration of breastfeeding.

Perhaps more breastfeeding women's groups are all we need, as it is difficult to know when a one-off celebration of breastfeeding would be best held. Having a group of experienced breastfeeding women turn up after the birth to share their knowledge with you would certainly put a stop to your babymoon, although it might help you have a good breast feeding experience in the early days of your baby's life. And waiting for your celebration until you were ready to wean would render the sharing of knowledge which tends to be a part of the gathering of women for these kind of rituals fairly defunct by then. Having said that, weaning parties might become the place to be if Western Governments recognised the massive value of breast milk in the economy and sent all mothers a bottle of champagne for every month they had breastfed their baby (and an extra magnum for women who had breastfed twins), to arrive on the day the mother and her baby decided to wean. This, coupled with a free babysitting service on an evening of the woman's choice, might then enable women to realise that their breasts have the same power as Hera's, and would probably encourage women to understand the sacredness and worth of their breasts more than any guilt-inducing poster campaign ever could.

Chapter 19

Cycling On

I've been thinking a lot about tangents while looking over the conversations I've had with some of the women whose experiences are in these pages. Each time I speak to a woman, I hear a new set of stories, and every single one of those stories is far more detailed, complex and rich than anything I could write about here. The stories in each individual woman's life, which often need to be told over and over again, form patterns; journeys begun and never finished, circles which complete years after they first started, spirals so complex they make DNA look simple. As I said in Chapter 1, with a remit to write about women's cycles, it wasn't my plan to write about women's sexuality, women's work, women's life journeys, women's experiences of abuse, the best and worst moments in women's lives. But these issues were all intertwined in the lives of the women I talked to. While books have a limit to the number of words you can write, and subjects you can cover, there are no word limits to women's stories.

Yet how many of those stories are heard?

I mean, *really* heard?

This is one example of a short exchange with Grace, a woman in her fifties who had recently extricated herself from a long-term relationship with an abusive partner. We were talking about one thing, when Grace began to talk about a different area (which later turned out to be a key point in the discussion). As soon as she realised, she had moved off the subject, Grace suddenly stopped. I was quiet for a minute, to give her time to think, and then she said:

Grace: "Oh, no, I'm going off on a tangent again, sorry..."
Sara: "No, it's fine, what you're saying is really interesting... You go off on tangents if you like..."

Grace: "I was always told how bad I was at going off on tangents... 'I wish you'd get to the bloody point', he'd always say, but I always found it hard to do that."

This wasn't an isolated comment; other women brought up the same thing, and the idea of wanting to "be heard", and wanting to "be allowed to process" certainly wasn't limited to women who had experienced abusive relationships;

"Wow, no-one's ever asked me about that before." (Belinda, who then went on to talk excitedly about the topic in question for fifteen minutes, before saying how glad she was that she had been able to, *"get that off my chest".*)

"We don't ... we don't really talk about some of these things, do we? ... But it is nice to be asked."

(Carolyn)

"I wish I could talk like this to my partner, and have him listen like this. He always says I go round and round too much"

(Emma)

I am, by the way, not the world's best listener. I try hard when I am interviewing people to stay focused on what they are saying, but I have to confess that sometimes my mind wanders off on tangents, often triggered by something they have just said, and I often have to fight back the desire to interrupt with a comment of my own. The point is, therefore, not about me, but, as so many researchers have found, about the fact that some women don't get listened to as much as they would like to be. Couple this with the realisation that many women truly enjoy the opportunity to process their thoughts as they arise ~ which is, more often than not, in non-logical order ~ and we have two big issues about how some women want to be heard when they are talking about their spirals.

Let's look first at the some of the issues around "being heard". In Chapter 7, I talked about the work of Mary Field Belenky and her colleagues, who looked at 'women's ways of knowing'. As before, they showed that a few women, often the youngest and most deprived, were "silent", feeling they had no voice. It struck me while I was talking to the women I inter-viewed that all of us, at any depth of understanding about knowledge, might still have an aspect of the silent woman inside us. Even those women who teach or speak to large groups of people for a living, and are listened to a lot in some areas of their life, talk about not being heard in other ways. As we cycle on and grow, we listen to others, and, if we have children, we listen to them, but who listens to us?

I find it interesting that, if you put the phrase "women's voices" into an Internet search engine, you will get a good-sized list of websites run by women who are trying to make a space for other women to be listened to. There are sites for hearing the voices (which is something of a misnomer as, like in this book, the women's words are often in print) of women from various cultural and ethnic groups, for hearing the voices of women who have sex with women, and the voices of women who lived and died before they knew that their words would one day be available for others to read on the Internet. If, on the other hand, you put "men's voices" into a search engine, you'll get a couple of sites trying to do a similar thing for men, and a lot of sites for music and choirs.

Our society has a long history of not recording and not hearing women's voices and women's stories. Where they have been recorded, they are often the voices and stories of the most privileged woman in a society. Historically, if you were a woman who became well known, or you were a woman in a position of power (or perhaps a woman married to a man in a position of power), your words might have been recorded for posterity. Yet even talent wasn't a guaranteed way of being heard; some women writers had to use male names to get their word into print. With this having been the norm for so many generations, no wonder so many women today feel they are not heard.

If we then move on to the ways in which women think, know and process, there is a general perception (although, of course, it is much more complex than this) that men process things in linear ways, and women process things in more circular, spiral, meandering, tangential ways. I asked my partner about this, to get a male perspective. He knows I like to be listened to when I am 'processing', yet often finds it hard to do this. (Sometimes he tries to put the TV on with the sound down in the background, so he can watch something while he 'listens', which just about drives me nuts!) I asked him why he found it so hard to simply listen to me when I want to share and process my thoughts out loud with him. In response, he immediately drew a series of pictures of this (curiously enough, in the dust on the TV screen!), while he explained what was going on for him, and I've reproduced them here (Figure 1).

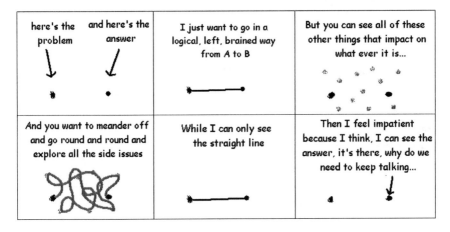

Figure 1.

Of course, there is another way of seeing this picture: while Figure 1 shows one male perspective on the issue, a possible female response to the same issue is shown in Figure 2.

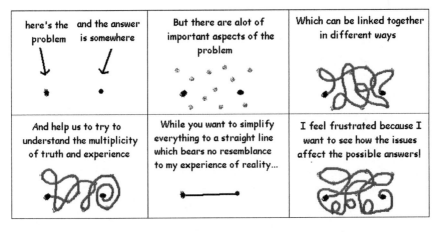

Figure 2.

While there are lots of other depictions of this process, for some people, one of these arguments might be more familiar than the other. I know that other women process things in different ways, as I am sure is the case for other men, and I am certainly not convinced that seeing this as either bipolar or entirely gender-based is helpful. Yet in some circles, we hear more about how difficult it is for men to deal with women spiralling off on tangents, while we hear less about how hard it is to be a woman in a society which is still primarily based on the idea that thought is (or, at least, should be) logical and linear. But other people have started to talk about how society is still more focused on linear ways of knowing, and think about what we might be able to do to redress the balance. In actuality, this debate goes much deeper, and links with questions about reality itself, with whether the world is based on causal relationships and certainties, on multiple possibilities, on a combination of these, or on something else entirely. Some people continue to look to classical science for certainty, while others argue that doubt, inconsistency and multiple possibilities are at the very heart of it all.

I have found previously, when studying (female) midwives, that women's stories are immensely important as a way of knowing:

> *"Midwives commonly use stories of their own and birthing women's experiences as evidence in practice. Midwives tell stories as a fundamental part of their "being with" women, often to help the woman to gain trust in her own body and her ability to birth. Ina May Gaskin (personal correspondence, 1999) describes the way in which she and the midwives she works with tell women experiencing long labours the story of Pamela, one of their colleagues, who was herself in labour for three days. On occasion they ask Pamela to come and see the labouring woman so that she can see for herself that Pamela survived the experience."*
>
> (Wickham 2003: 163–4)

I have watched how different groups of midwives interact, and how they learn by sharing stories and experience. Often, one midwife will begin a conversation by asking a question, perhaps about the use of a particular technique, or what other midwives would do in a given scenario. More often than not, one of the other midwives in the group will take the lead in responding with details and stories about her experience in the area. The rest of the midwives will join in the conversation at different points; some will support the aspects of this midwife's understanding which has also been their own experience, and some will share stories of their own where their experience has been different. The conversation will spiral around, going off on tangents, perhaps returning to the original question, or perhaps going off in a completely different direction. The midwives I interviewed in this instance were those who work outside of "the system" in their country, so I cannot claim this is true of all midwives, or all women, but it was extremely rarely that I would find a woman/midwife who wasn't comfortable with this spiralling, tangential kind of conversation.

As we spiral on through our lives, our stories become more and more varied, deeper and richer and often, I would say, more interesting with time. As we experience more of life, we have more to tell, which makes it paradoxical that some of the older women I talked to seem to feel less heard, and less understood than when they were younger. I talked in Chapter 6 about how interesting and useful it would be for young girls to hear the stories of older women; I suspect it would be just as empowering for the older women who were able to have their stories heard.

We continue to see new and improved TV game shows which test factual knowledge, physical dexterity and linear thinking, again enforcing the idea that these are the most valuable skills and ways of knowing. I can't wait for the first TV show which is consistently won by women, at least initially, because it tests the things that women tend to be better at. Who will be the first to offer a prize for "the number of interesting tangents one can go-off on in one conversation", for "the longest conversation between two or more people which eventually comes back to the point where it started", or for "the most interesting thing I have learned in my life, and how I got there"? It would be great to see a talk show where the presenter wasn't so preoccupied with cutting people off because their story had gone on for too long, or where members of the audience didn't shout over each other, but really listened to other points of view and then discussed them in a reasonable manner. But, in the meantime, even if just thought about whether and how we could listen more to each other, it would be a start.

Chapter 20

Celebrating the Matriarch

In writing about women's lives and the different archetypes, or inner patterns, which women might experience at different stages of their life-spiral, Elizabeth Davis and Carol Leonard used the three aspects of the 'triple Goddess' to represent different stages of women's lives; maiden, mother and crone. It is easy to see the correlations between the maiden and menarche, between the mother and childbirth and between the crone (which, in this context, is considered a very positive word) and menopause. Yet they found the need to consider another phase in women's life cycles, because, for many women, there was such a space between becoming a mother and reaching menopause.

Davis and Leonard called the archetype which represents this almost-forgotten phase "the matriarch" and describe her as follows:

> "She is us, when childbearing urges begin to wane, when careers are well established and a sense of mastery comes upon us. Not yet in menopause, still beset with worldly responsibilities but longing for something more, the Matriarch rekindles the passions and dreams of youth, and may pick up broken threads of spiritual pursuits with new intensity and direction."
>
> (Davis and Leonard 1996: 4)

I explored with a few of the women I talked to what was happening for them in this space, and whether this time was characterised by anything in particular:

> "I'm 45 now and I feel as though I am peri-menopausal, my menstrual cycle is a bit more erratic etc ... and it does feel as

though I have made some quite big changes in my life over the last few years. One of those has been starting a PhD, it feels as though I am growing into my academic career ... At the same time I have felt a real need to do more midwifery practice and have joined the midwifery bank and am now 'midwifing' a friend who is planning to have her third babe at home in July. Over the last year ... and this has been the most surprising for me ... I have also felt a really strong need to use my hands to be creative and have taken up knitting again after a gap of more than twenty years! So, yes, it does feel as though it is a time of growth, e.g. the PhD, but also a time of grounding, the hands-on midwifery, and creativity, the knitting."

(Monika)

"I found the wheel of archetypes really helpful in recognising what I was experiencing. Growth is continuous, as a woman, and the time between children leaving and menopause has personally been particularly satisfying for me. But [it's] mainly because I had already been a physical mother ... I don't believe this would have been possible without giving birth and mothering, for me, anyway. The wheel enables me to look forward to further growth and experience without any feeling of loss ... while really experiencing the present."

(Genevieve)

Davis and Leonard proposed the idea that, on their wheel, each of the archetypes 'faced' another one and could be compared to it. Their matriarch archetype faced the 'maiden' archetype, which represents the transformation form child to woman through puberty and the menarche. I found it very interesting, then, when a couple of the women I talked to (who, unlike Genevieve, hadn't read Davis and Leonard's book) compared their transition towards menopause with their experiences as teenagers:

"I keep wondering if it's possible that there's a transition which happens, like the one I feel is happening in me, that's similar to the one we experience when we're a teenager? I don't know, but it sort of feels like it's a similar time."

(Anastacia)

*"I'm not at the menopause yet, but my periods are changing,
and I suppose I'm getting there ~ I feel like a teenager again ~
I have moods, I want to go to my bedroom and sulk, and I feel
sometimes [that] I'm not in control of my emotions."*

(Poppy)

Somehow, I doubt that many women who are nearing menopause would want to be compared to teenage girls outside of this context, not least because our culture already views menopausal women in a somewhat negative light, and this might be construed by some people as a further slight. Our culture sometimes seems to make more of the actual events of our lifespirals than the transitions between them, which may be one reason why, in recent times, we are only just beginning to work on finding space for the women who are on this journey. For instance, it sometimes seems that we give more attention to the actual birth of a baby than we do to the pregnancy or the early mothering period.

If we consider the actual definitions of the terms 'menarche' and 'menopause', we find that they refer to fairly specific events; the first menstrual period, and the last menstrual period. Yet both of these may be difficult to determine as an actual event; a woman's first period may be little more than a couple of drops of pinkish blood, or a little cramp with no bleeding at all, and a woman won't know which period was her last until she has lived a couple of years without another one. Indeed, some women might think that a particular period they experienced was their last, only to find that after a year of no periods at all, they suddenly and unexpectedly have another one.

The reality of menarche, menopause and other 'events' in women's lifespirals is that they are journeys, which may take several years to fully complete. Perhaps we need to move away from the medical definitions of these words and create a new language that better describes our experiences? As with any good journey, the experiences that we have in between the actual events and excursions may be more interesting than the excursions themselves! Charles De Lint, one of my favourite fiction authors, often says in his books that the 'in-between' is where magic occurs. And in-between is certainly the place where the women experiencing the matriarch archetype seem to find themselves.

Where is the sacred space for the middle-aged woman? She may be busy working hard and successfully in her career, supporting the young women and men who were once her children but who have now gone away to study or start families of their own. She may be at home, having waved her children goodbye as they went into the world, wondering what will happen in her life next. She may be making plans to study or take a 'gap year' herself, or she may, as is increasingly common, still be at home with young children, having started her own family later in life. She may be alone, experiencing a life of solitude, or have a life so filled with happenings that there is little time to think. She may be joyously happy with the choices she has made and the opportunities she has encountered, or she may have unfulfilled dreams which, every so often, creep into her thoughts.

Wherever and whoever she is, she may be on a journey that isn't visible from the outside. The in-between-ness may be soaking into her pores, causing her to enrol for a PhD or pick up her knitting again, like Monika, or, then again, perhaps she will not experience the in-between at all. Is it a coincidence that a fair number of women reach this stage and then decide they are not, after all, happy with their marriage? Were Shirley Valentine and Thelma and Louise exploring the in-between?

Perhaps this is one of the stages of the lifespiral where the spiral might look more like a labyrinth, full of knots and puzzles, but with a way into the centre, which you can always reach if you walk for long enough. Diane Schaper and Carole Ann Camp suggest that a labyrinth is more than a maze, because you can explore complexity without ever getting lost:

> "You are always on the path leading into or out of the centre. One
> finds the centre if one walks the path. A labyrinth is like a maze
> with a certain answer ... if we but walk the path, we get home."
> (Schaper and Camp 2000: 2)

While there may be commonalities in our 'centres', which we have yet to explore, perhaps during the matriarchal years we each have an opportunity to walk the labyrinth of our own lives; reframing the old, choosing the new, tidying our metaphorical cupboards to revive the dreams we haven't yet lived, putting away those which once seemed important but whose importance has now faded with time, and exploring the magic of the in-between.

Chapter 21

Towards the Menopause

In the same way that menstruating women have, in the relatively recent history of some cultures, come to be seen as 'dirty', a menopausal woman in modern Western society may be seen as 'past her prime'. For many women, the menopause ~ like menstruation and birth ~ has become a physical, medical event, perhaps something to be dreaded. It has become associated with women growing older, coming to the end of our fertility, experiencing the loss of our children as they begin to make their own way in the world ~ all of which are viewed by many as things to fear, rather than relish. One group of women, when I asked them to think about some of the words which relate to the menopause (without giving them any more information or suggestions about this), produced the following list:

Hormonal	Osteoporosis	Past your sell-by-date
Wrinkly	New horizons	Sexually incompetent
Had it	Moody	Dried up
Barren	Hot flashes	HRT
Hairy	Irregular periods	The change
Middle age	Low self-esteem	Turkey neck
Crinkly	Dry vagina	Old
Finished	Infertile	Wisdom
Prune-like	The sweats	Past it

We then looked more closely at these 27 words and saw that they fell into several categories:

- Six related to age, mostly in ways that the women in the group felt were negative.

- Six related to dryness or wrinkling of the body.
- Four could be considered physical symptoms or problems.
- Three could be considered psychological or emotional symptoms or problems.
- Two could be considered positive ("wisdom" and "new horizons").
- The group felt that "hairy", "HRT", "the change" and "hormonal" didn't fall into any of these categories and might, depending on the individual woman, be seen as positive, negative or neutral ~ although I should add that only two of the women present didn't think that "hairy" had negative connotations.

I wonder how many women nearing the menopause in Western society are influenced by the general attitude to menopause, and by the words and concepts which are associated with this spiral? How many women see menopause as a sign that they are becoming "past it", or that they are "drying up"? At almost any stage of our lives we may find our relationships and lives changing in subtle or substantial ways, yet women nearing the menopause may see these things as confirmation that, as Lottie noted, *'it's all downhill from here'*. Seeking medical advice and taking hormones and drugs to lessen these feelings and symptoms may seem the only way forward.

But in many other societies and groups menopausal women are seen as the wisest of all people, those who are given roles such as teacher, counsellor, lawmaker and judge. Their wisdom, experience and knowledge is respected and revered. Women of the Seneca tribe who are nearing menopause consult with other older women and choose a subject that they will then teach others, and women of some Jewish and Native American traditions mark their menopause by changing their names (Davis 2000). For many women, menopause is an exciting journey, which leads them on to new adventures they never thought possible. As Margaret Mead famously said ...

> *"There is no more creative force in the world than the menopausal woman with zest."*

The term 'menopause' was first used in 1862, from the Greek words for 'month' and 'cessation'. At around the same time, the menopause began to be seen by Western doctors as a crisis that caused many diseases. This may have stemmed in part from the earlier belief held by doctors that the uterus wandered around the woman's body, causing mayhem as it went. They believed that if the wandering uterus reached the woman's brain, it caused hysteria ~ it is no coincidence that the word hysterical has the same root as words like hysterectomy. Women were seen to be most at risk of this disease if they had acted indiscreetly, gained too much education or enjoyed sex more than they should! However, even at this time, some people also noticed the menopause was a time of increased vigour, optimism and physical beauty.

Nowadays, Western medicine has moved away from the tendency to see menopause as the cause of disease, but now sometimes classes it as a disease in itself, despite the fact that this is a perfectly normal spiral in women's lives. (In fact, it is the woman who did not go through the menopause, and carried on menstruating until her seventies who would be atypical, and thus worthy of note). It would be unfair to say that the idea that menopause is a disease is the opinion of every doctor: some enlightened doctors criticise their colleagues for the unnecessary ~ but all too often routine ~ removal of women's organs and their insistence on seeing the menopause as a medical and negative event. Yet some of the woman I spoke to felt quite strongly that their 'change of life' was viewed as a problem, when all they wanted was information, or reassurance that their experiences were 'normal':

> [What I was offered was] HRT or a long walk home ... When I
> said I was worried about HRT and didn't want to [take it] unless
> I really had to, he wasn't interested. What I wanted, though ...
> I just wanted to know more.
>
> (Fiona)

> The first time I went I felt they weren't listening, they
> didn't think this stuff was a problem. The second time it
> was like, if it's a problem then this is what you take. [There
> was] no discussion of the side effects though ... that's what
> worried me.
>
> (Carolyn)

Of course, women have all kinds of different attitudes towards menopause:

> *It didn't bother me, not really, my periods stopped and I carried on. I didn't really think about it.*
>
> (Clare)

> *I did stop and think ... what if ... you know, what if I'd wanted more babies, it was probably too late now. Then I'd think, NO! It's OK.*
>
> (Fiona)

> *It was bloody miserable. I thought I hated my periods, but I think at one time I thought I'd rather have had them back than all of those hot flashes.*
>
> (Ruth)

One group of women who I talked to together found a metaphor which worked well for them:

Izzy: *It feels to me like a sea, yeah that's a good way of describing it ... the whole thing I mean, over time. I'm swimming around in the menopause sea* (the whole group starts to laugh, as Izzy is now pulling faces and making swimming movements) *and sometimes it's calm and sometimes it's a storm, but usually if I float I'm OK. When I struggle with it, I've learned ... when I struggle ... that's when it's harder. You sort of have to let it go and surrender to it.*
Carolyn: *Don't you ever wish you had a boat though?!*
Izzy: *Well I suppose I could get on the HRT boat ... have a herbal life raft, but ... I suppose ... I rather like knowing I'm swimming it myself...*
Pat: *Well I'd rather go on a cruise than swim!*
Carolyn: *The menopause cruise, that'd be a good brand name for HRT!*
Sue: *Shall we try and market it?*
Izzy: *Yeah, but that's the thing ... I know you're not all into it, but you'd miss all the fun swimming!*

At the end of this discussion, we had discovered that Izzy gained huge satisfaction from swimming alone in the menopause sea and Pat was very happy on her HRT cruise until the whole thing was over. (This reminded me a bit of the contrast between the women who gain a huge sense of their own power from birthing without drugs, and those who want to have an epidural no matter what anyone says about the joy of birth.) Sue hadn't experienced any real problems that she felt she needed a life raft for, and Carolyn felt she was just about coping by using vitamins and eating lots of phytoestrogen-rich foods but was glad she knew there were other alternatives. Sarah, who was at the beginning of her menopause journey, said she needed to go away and meditate some more on the swimming decision, as she thought she might try to practice ways to float, so she wouldn't ever have to struggle...

Professionals who see menopausal women are probably just as varied in their attitudes to this as women are themselves, yet there is indeed a significant and powerful school of thought in Western culture which views menopause as a deficiency disease, like diabetes. While individual doctors may not subscribe to this belief, this school of thought may impact on the way many women feel about their bodies at this time.

People who have "deficiency diseases" like diabetes are noted to have lower levels of a substance (in the case of diabetes, it is the hormone insulin) in their bodies than most people. Consequently, they may experience symptoms that arise from insulin deficiency. This deficiency is treated by altering the person's diet, checking the levels of the hormone through blood tests and sometimes through the use of synthetic insulin. In the same way, menopause has come to be seen in some circles as a "deficiency disease"; where the deficiency is in the hormones (oestrogens and progesterone) whose levels begin to fall at this time. Just as the diabetic may be seen to need insulin (although it should be noted that some people suggest that at least some forms of this could be treated differently), the menopausal woman may be seen as needing synthetic forms of the hormones whose levels have dropped in her body.

One of the "facts" cited to support this argument is where people suggest that, in ancient societies, women did not live past the age of about forty or fifty, and so would have died before reaching the menopause. If you believe this argument, it then becomes logical to assume that the menopause is a mistake; it was never meant to happen to our bodies, and therefore the replacement of our hormones with synthetic hormones is a good thing.

Unfortunately, it is very difficult to know whether this "fact" is true or not. We know very little about ancient societies, and how long people lived, not least because the fossil record for human ancestors is so sparse. While we know that people who lived a couple of hundred years ago in the West had more ill-health than we do now, this was probably as much a result of the crowded living and the effects of industrialisation as anything else. It is naïve to think that every society before us must have been less healthy than our own ~ societies living before pollution, man-made disease and unhealthy diets may have contained many people living to ripe old ages!

Taking into account what we currently know about these issues, while I can't 'prove' the argument that women were meant to live past the menopause, there is equally no substance to the argument that they weren't. The truth is, we just don't know, although, as will be discussed in the next chapter, there are some interesting arguments about whether future generations may benefit from our living beyond menopause. When we face an absence of sound knowledge and 'not-knowingness' in an area such as this, our attitudes are often then based on what we choose to believe. In the case of menopause, we are free to choose our own beliefs from the range which encompasses, on the one hand, the idea that menopause is an unhealthy, unnecessary and unpleasant disease and, on the other, the idea that the menopause is a spiral that is a natural, healthy and wondrous journey in a woman's life.

The menopause spiral has become almost totally defined in the Western written word as a physical journey, perhaps partly as another result of our culture's emphasis on the physical, and on the health of the body. Even the sources of information which go on to tell you about supplements and other ways of "managing" menopause without HRT begin with the physical symptoms of menopause, the causes of these and the effects they can have on the body.

While the bottom line for me with all of these things is that women should be able to make their own choices, and not be hounded into choosing the current social or medical trend, or the suggestions of books like this one, I do feel there are aspects of the menopause, in common with the other spirals of women's lives, that aren't currently well-known, and that women have a right to the information on this side of the picture. In fact, there are plenty of women who think that there are positive advantages to our decreasing hormone levels at this time, as the next chapter will explore ...

Chapter 22

Positive Menopause

If we look at what actually happens during the menopause, we can get some idea of what the advantages might be. As we do this, it seems to be really important to pick up the point made by several of the women I talked to that the menopause isn't usually something that happens overnight ~ it is a journey. Like puberty, for most women, it comes gradually. At first, a woman might wonder if her menopause journey is beginning, only to realise that a skipped period was due to stress, or a "hot flash" was actually the beginning of her having the flu. Or she might experience changes which she puts down to stress, only later to recognize that they were the first signs of her menopause. Like any other journey, once the menopause starts, there may be times when it seems more intense, and times when women might forget they are on a journey at all.

The language we use around this time is interesting ~ and often quite vague. However, while vague language is sometimes used because we do not know enough to have clarified exactly what we mean, in the case of menopause it may (whether accidentally or by design) link with the imprecise and personal nature of the journey itself. We talk about women being "pre-menopausal", "menopausal" and "post-menopausal", yet in one sense we are pre-menopausal for most of our lives, until we know for sure we have reached menopause. Strictly speaking, "menopause" itself (especially when it is used in a medical context, almost as a diagnosis) can only be established in retrospect, as it refers to a time when periods have stopped ~ and, as before, many women experience a time when they think that they have reached menopause only to find that, after six months without a period, they then have three in quick succession. Although in medical circles people also use the term "peri-menopause" (which literally means "around the time of menopause"), this term does not tend to be used much by women themselves. I often wonder which generation of women will create new words for menopause, in the way that the American midwives in the nineteen-sixties counterculture crafted new words around birth when the older, medical words didn't fit their perceptions of this journey.

On a physical level, the journey of menopause is said to happen as the levels of some of our female hormones are beginning to decrease. During peri-menopause the levels of different kinds of oestrogens in a woman's body begin to fall, which causes periods to become more irregular, sometimes lighter (although sometimes much heavier too) and then eventually stop. Levels of the hormone progesterone also decrease. The lowered levels of these hormones can lead to some of the changes women experience in their bodies at this time, although it is also important to note that many men who are the same age as menopausal women experience some of the same kinds of changes. While some people debate whether there is a 'male menopause', it seems far more likely to me that there is a blurring between changes that are a result of altered hormone levels and changes that simply go along with growing older. Coney goes even further than this in suggesting that:

> *"The so-called menopausal syndrome is an unscientific mish-mash of fact, fallacy and prejudice. Menopause has become a catch-all, a dump-bin for everything that is happening to mid-life women. The medical menopause is something of a con."*
>
> (Coney 1995: 94)

> *"Women need to reject an ideology which leads to a preoccupation with ill-health and which inculcates a sense of precious mortality. Instead of 'living gingerly', mid-life women should insist on their right to live life with verve, gusto and spice."*
>
> (Coney 1995: 277)

But we have still only really discussed what is happening on a physical level. If you buy a book about the menopause in a high street shop, or visit one of the numerous web sites about the menopause, the physical aspects of menopause are precisely where the information (and sometimes misinformation) will start. But, as the words of the women in the previous chapter showed, exploring how women feel about the menopause can raise some very interesting issues. Some women also feel it is also important to explore the spirituality of the menopause journey:

> *"In menopause, I am certain that we have the chance to merge with the greater self, that one, that reflective visionary one, who has been running along beside us all our lives long."*
>
> (Estés 1996: 101–2)

The social aspects of menopause are equally fascinating. Some of the older women I spoke to told me that they suffered (their word, not mine) their menopause alone, with only the occasional shared glance or rolling of their eyes towards another woman of similar age or experience to communicate that they were going through a difficult time. This couldn't contrast more with the idea of a "croning" party or ritual, which, like a "first period" party, enables a woman to celebrate this rite of passage socially, with other women of all ages:

> *"Most menopause rituals naturally incorporate practices for letting go of the past and welcoming new responsibilities. For example, women may gather around a fire (or a symbolic candle) and take turns, one by one, giving up some fear, resentment, or self-limiting belief to be consumed by the flame. If the fire is large enough, each woman can throw in a token of her surrender ~ a piece of wood, paper, cloth, or other symbolic item. As each woman takes her turn, she speaks of her deepest lesson in life, and of that which she still intends to accomplish."*
>
> (Davis 2000: 185)

Croning, like the idea of celebrating our daughters' first periods, is an entirely personal preference. I have one friend who is desperate for her periods to stop because she can't wait for her croning ritual; she is very excited, and enjoys thinking about what it might include. And I have another who once told me that, if I even thought about holding a croning ritual for her, she would never speak to me again! There are always going to be some women who hate the idea of 'going public' with aspects of their journey, and some women who enjoy nothing better than sharing their experiences of that journey. Incidentally, for those women in the second group, Leonard offers the following advice on dealing with hot flashes:

"You could yell, "I'm hotter than a red-assed bee!" That's what my grandmother did every time she had a hot flash. (I am entirely serious)."

(Leonard 1999: 43)

But are there other social advantages to menopause? In stark contrast to the view (challenged in the previous chapter) that menopause is a mistake brought on by our living longer than we are meant to, new research provides evidence that menopause may bring distinct advantages to the woman as well as the social group (Lahdenperä et al 2004). Lahdenperä and her colleagues suggest that the 'life-history theory' (the idea that we were not supposed to live beyond our reproductive lifespan) is not initially as improbable as we might like to think, as it is certainly true that the majority of animals do not live beyond the point where they become unable to reproduce. They then go on the discuss the main challenge to the 'life-history theory', the 'grandmother theory', which proposed that there was an advantage to the whole social group where grandmothers stopped having their own babies and helped bring up their own children's babies, which would improve the survival rates (on the basis that grandmothers are very experienced and knowledgeable about bringing up children).

In order to try to strengthen or refute this theory, they analysed eighteenth and nineteenth century records of births and deaths in Canadian and Finnish farming communities, where families tend to have close ties. In both countries, the older a woman was when she died, the more grandchildren she tended to have. (This includes grandchildren born after her death; it was not simply that she died before the later grandchildren were born.) Their data also showed that the presence of a living, post-menopausal grandmother in a family decreased the spacing between children in a family (perhaps because they were able to offer the kind of help that enabled the younger women to contemplate having another child more quickly) and increased the likelihood that the children would survive after the age of two (when breastfeeding generally stopped and the grandmother was perhaps more involved in their care).

The researchers aren't saying that the 'grandmother effect' is the only reason we experience menopause, but they do conclude that this effect could account for the fact that human women can live for a long time after they stop being able to reproduce. One of the menopausal women I talked to certainly felt there was something interesting about the way we are more likely to listen to the advice given by older women:

> *"I think it's difficult when you're start going through it because you sort of lose your own confidence ... having been a very confident woman you start to swing and think 'oh, you can't do that'. On the other hand it's great fun because people expect you be that bit more batty and outspoken. Then there is that feeling that because you're older you've experienced more life and looked at it longer ... that what you say is worth considering, not necessarily following, but considering."*
>
> (Frances)

The implications of us not having a menopause are also interesting... If we were still able to conceive and birth babies into our seventies and eighties (as, indeed, many men can father babies until this time), we would have little time or energy to enjoy our grandchildren as we would still be preoccupied with raising our own children. Our children, however, would be far more likely to have to suffer the loss of their parents ~ and to have to deal with all of the emotional, social and practical implications of this loss ~ at a relatively early age. Instead, Lahdenperä's research suggests that this benefit declines when a woman's children reach menopause, and they do show a correlation between women reaching menopause and the death of their own mothers. They hypothesise that this might be because the younger women, who have now reached menopause themselves, are able to take over the tasks of helping their own offspring to raise children.

It would seem that the menopause journey is far more complex, and far more important than we have previously realised. For several years, I have facilitated menopause workshops for women who wanted to explore these issues further and, after my friend Lorna (of marathon running fame) studied "birth art", I began to offer women the chance to paint their menopause experience during workshops. I'm not an art therapist, and I made it very clear that we weren't going to go really deep with this, but even doing this at a basic level seemed to work really well. Some of the women said they felt freer to 'play' than they had for a long time, and almost all of the women I have done this with have learned something about their menopause that they didn't know before. If more of us could find more ways to play, then perhaps we would find out even more about the positive aspects of menopause.

As I have said before, women have been socialised for decades into believing that their bodies are inferior, and that they are not very good at doing their 'jobs' of giving birth, feeding babies or taking us into old age. Our society tends to see menopause as a 'bad' thing; at best an irritation in women's lives, at worst a time of turmoil and trauma which impacts on women and those around them.

Every one of us can make the choice not to believe these things. I don't personally see how the negative beliefs that are held around menopause are of any use to women; I don't feel that they are accurate. I believe there are positive advantages to going on this journey and to being post-menopausal. I have seen many women 'find themselves' through their menopause, sometimes because they suffered symptoms, and sought help for those, they then met other women who helped them to empower them-selves and learn more about their bodies. I have met women for whom the menopause was the trigger they needed to re-train, to learn new skills, to begin to travel the world, and to find a new lease of life.

When I talk to post-menopausal women, they often tell me how liberated they feel. One of my friends tells me that, until she reached menopause, she never realised just how much her life and her decisions were governed by the hormones of her menstrual cycle. This was fine while she was growing and having her family, but she was ready to leave that behind as she travelled through menopause. Another friend told me, on my thirtieth birthday, that she wished she had known when she was thirty that there were some things she couldn't possibly know until she reached the age of sixty. It seems the wisdom that came after the menopause for women in ancient societies is still alive and well today, and begging to be grasped by those women who have reached "a certain age" ~ although I feel the age itself is actually less certain than the fact that all women have the potential for incredible growth through this spiral.

How different our society would be if it was governed ~ even in part ~ by menopausal women, who shared their knowledge and wisdom with younger women and men, who passed on their crafts and their experience, who made the laws of our countries and counselled the needy. I imagine the world would be very different. At the very least, I hope for a society where the majority of menopausal women are aware of the range of choices available to them, and where they grasp their menopausal zest in both hands and run with it!

Chapter 23

A Sourcebook of Menopausal Choices

As in Chapter 10, Susun Weed's model seems a good way to me of laying out the options we have during the menopausal spiral, whether in seeking a cure for particular symptoms which are posing a problem, or because we want to further explore what this journey means for us. I have listed in here some possibilities at each stage, moving from the steps with the least potential for harm and side effects to the more invasive therapies. Again, I have used the same key to enable you to see where the information comes from and make your own assessment of it. As a reminder:

《 ～ denotes information which has come from women's experience, and which has worked for at least one woman whom I have talked to.

☐ ～ denotes information which came from at least one research study of reasonable quality (and which was not sponsored by the company who manufactures the product being sold!).

✱ ～ denotes information which came from at least one research study where the quality could have been better or where the company which sells the product sponsored the research but where the results may still be worth considering.

○ ～ denotes information which has come from another source (e.g. something somebody heard but hasn't tried themselves, a suggestion made in an article but not referenced, a web site which appears to be based on giving information rather than selling products, or from a letter or email sent to me by someone I haven't talked to personally).

Some people describe menopause as the reverse of puberty and, indeed, several of the suggestions in here parallel some of the suggestions that have been made in the chapters exploring moon lodging and menstrual choices and remedies. But I'm not convinced that it is always ideal to view the spiral of menopause in this way ~ although, as above, some women do report feeling "like teenagers again" or having temper tantrums and mood swings when they are on the journey of menopause! There might be loose parallels between the ideas of periods starting and periods stopping, and in hormones increasing during the first, and decreasing during the second. But we are only really beginning to listen for, and hear, women's voices on the subject of what these experiences are like; if we can hold a space for long enough, without trying to pre-empt the answer we will find out far more...

Step 0: Do nothing

- Just as there is benefit in resting at certain times of a woman's menstrual cycle, some women also benefit enormously from resting at different times of their menopause journey, either at the times of the month when they do have periods, or when they would have had a period, or during the full moon, or simply whenever they feel the need. ☽
- Given that many women of menopausal age still have responsibilities, whether through family, work or in other areas of their life, many of the things that have already been said about finding time (and allowing ourselves time) to moon lodge are equally true of menopause. For a few women, regular phone-free sessions, long bubble baths, peaceful evenings with meditation tapes or solitary walks in the woods have made all the difference. ☽
- Trying to 'float' with symptoms such as hot flashes (in the way that Izzy described in Chapter 21) can reduce their effect. ☽

Step 1: Collect information

- There are simply tens of books and hundreds of web sites about different aspects of the menopause: you may want to find out a bit about whether the author of the book or owner of the web site shares your philosophy on this, or look at all kinds of information in order to decide what your own philosophy is...
- Some women who have experienced severe problems with hot flashes, have found it was helpful to keep a diary. This has helped them to

identify ~ and then perhaps avoid ~ any triggers which seem to be linked to their hot flashes. Some women find their hot flashes are linked to certain types of food or stressful events in their lives.
- There is also huge value in talking to other women and the number of menopause support groups, Internet newsgroups and workshops on this topic is growing daily.

Step 2: Engage the energy

During the menopause spiral, energy can be engaged for a number of reasons; to better understand what is happening, to deal with specific issues or symptoms that arise during the journey, or simply to be with ourselves on the journey. Some of the things that worked for the women I talked to include:

- Flower remedies. (
- Prayer, meditation, cultivating the stillness within. (
- Women's evenings in cosy places, with any combination of wine, chocolate, flowers, music, laughter, tears, cats, honesty, friendship, love... (
- If you need inspiration to begin talking with other women about the menopause, try writing the following sentences on pieces of card, and then letting each woman in turn pick it up, read it out and finish the sentence in her own words...
  - The thing I like most about the menopause is...
  - I knew I was on my menopausal journey when...
  - The most difficult aspect of menopause for me is...
  - The thing I wish I could tell all women about the menopause is...
  - The best book or article I ever read about the menopause is...
  - My favourite way of dealing with hot flashes is...
  - The part of the menopause I could really do without is...
  - The funniest thing about the menopause is...
  - When it comes to the menopause, I would tell young women that...
  - I think I will look back on my menopause and feel that...
  - The part of my menopausal journey I still need to complete is...
  - The thing I am most looking forward to after my menopause is...
- One woman I spoke to said the most helpful thing of all was, *"Allowing myself to cry ~ it took me more than fifty years not to feel guilty"* (

- Essential oils may also help, on both energetic and physical levels (both are discussed here, along with specific properties which you may want to look into further if you think they may be of help): ☾ ✱
  - Lavender is generally relaxing and calming. It can offer relief from pain, particularly that related to the uterus. However, it can bring on a period and sometimes increases vaginal bleeding.
  - Tangerine is a balancing oil and can help lift your mood. It can be used with lavender oil and is particularly pleasant when diffused in a room. All citrus oils can stain skin if exposed to sunlight, and may be irritating to some people's skin.
  - Geranium can also help lift your mood and provide relief from mild depression, and some therapists feel that it helps balance reproductive hormones.
  - Marjoram can be helpful for sleep problems such as insomnia.
  - Ylang ylang is a relaxing and balancing oil which also works well as an aphrodisiac! It can be combined with lavender, and/or geranium.
- Homeopathic remedies (though, as before, you need to find out what fits your personal situation). ☾ ✱
- Consider using craft skills you have (or might like to develop) to create something that symbolises your menopausal journey. Perhaps a cushion, quilt, skirt, hat, some jewellery, a pot, a garden, candles... ☾
- A significant number of the women I talked to had realised that there are at least three ways to look at the changes which take place in women's bodies at this time, whether they are linked with menopause or not. Option one is to see these changes as bad, and to focus on the negative implications (e.g. my hair is thinning and greying, my body is failing and I no longer fit modern society's ideal of youthful good looks and high energy levels). Option two is to be non-judgemental about the whole thing, and to simply notice that the changes are happening, but not to judge them as either positive or negative. Option three is to make an effort to "think positively" about these changes (I can enjoy sex more now. I don't have to worry about contraception and I am entering a new, wise and exciting phase of my life) and to focus on the "verve, gusto and spice"! ☾
- To paint your menopause, start with a big artist's pad (it can be one of the inexpensive kind, but bigger certainly seems to work better for

some women!), a couple of fat paintbrushes (because fat brushes prevent you from doing fine lines and therefore engage the right, intuitive side of your brain, rather than your left, logical side) a few poster paints and whatever old pots or cups you have for storing water or mixing paint to make different colours. Then, close your eyes for a minute, ask yourself for a picture of your menopause and, when you're ready, open your eyes and paint! When you've finished, you can see if it "says" anything to you that you didn't know: you might also want to try this with friends, because people often notice things in each others' pictures that they may not notice themselves. Some of the questions you can ask yourself about your picture are...

– What kind of journey is your menopause?
– Are you in the picture? Whereabouts? Is anyone else there?
– If you have painted a journey, how far along are you on the journey?
– If you have not painted a journey, where 'are' you in relation to your menopause?
– Does your picture tell you anything you didn't know about your journey, or about how you are feeling on it?

Step 3: Nourish and tonify

- You can nourish your body by wearing cotton clothing and using used cotton bed linen. Leave bedding loose so it can be easily removed at night. Dress in layers, which can easily be removed during the day. ☾
- If you experience vaginal dryness or itching, re-consider the kind of sanitary protection you are using when you bleed. Tampons tend to dry out the vagina even more, and the kind of sanitary towels that advertise 'super-absorbency' may contain chemicals or powders, which will draw moisture away from the skin. See Chapter 10 for other options. ☾
- Many sources suggest you cut down on stimulants such as cigarettes, caffeine and alcohol, which can make hot flashes worse. ☾ ☐ However, sometimes, these things can also make us feel a lot better, and, if this is the case for you, you may choose to celebrate that something works rather than making yourself feel guilty.
- Some foods actually ease menopausal symptoms, particularly those containing high levels of nutrients, such as fruits, vegetables, grains, legumes, nuts, seeds, bean and peas. The high fibre content of grains regulates hormone levels (particularly oestrogen) and whole

grains contain high levels of vitamins B and E which are critical for healthy hormone balance, regulation of oestrogen and can help reduce fatigue and depression. ❨ ☐

- Soybean-based products are among those which actually help reduce and prevent menopausal symptoms. (This may be why Japanese woman, who eat lots of soy and soy-derived products, have far fewer menopausal symptoms than their British and American sisters). ❨ ☐
- Other pulses (e.g. lentils, kidney, butter or black beans) are high in vitamin B complex, which is essential for a healthy liver. Liver function is important at the time of the menopause as the liver breaks down oestrogen. For this reason it can also be helpful to reduce the amount of fat and alcohol in your diet, as the metabolism of these substances can put extra strain on the liver. ❨ ☐
- Fat is not all bad ~ essential fatty acids (EFAs) can prevent inflammation, relieve tissue dryness and prevent symptoms of arthritis. They also assist in the production of prostaglandins, which stimulate the immune system and can help prevent some of the problems that lead to heart disease. Replacing animal fats with EFAs from seeds, seed oils, supplemented breakfast cereals or flax oil and evening primrose supplements can help ensure you will get enough 'good' fat. ❨ ☐
- Some women find they benefit from avoiding meat, or choosing organic meat, as some meat contains animal hormones that can exacerbate menopausal symptoms. Again, this is a personal issue, as some women find they feel better after eating meat. ❨
- Exercise can help keep the body supple during menopause, and is one of the best ways of preventing the possibility of osteoporosis. ❨ ☐
- Vitamin D is needed for bone regeneration, and it helps the body retain calcium. It is made in the skin, so the best source is exposure to sunlight.

Step 4: Stimulate/sedate

- A midwife friend of mine used to suggest to women that they stimulate their adrenal glands (which are involved in the production of reproductive hormones) to reduce hot flashes, either by alternating hot and cold (compresses or shower) or by asking a friend or partner to tap on them for a couple of minutes per day. ❨ ✱

- During a hot flash or sweat, some women find it helps to put the inside of their wrists and arms on a cold surface, or to put ice packs on them for a minute or so. ☾
- Acupuncture, homeopathy and/or massage can also be useful during menopause. ☾ ☐✱
- A number of herbs have been suggested to help relieve hot flashes, although some (marked with asterisks) contain high levels of oestrogen-like substances and need to be taken with care. This is the point in Weed's model where side effects and interactions can start to occur, so the following list includes ideas for research/discussion with a herbalist rather than suggestions for personal treatment:
  - Ginseng*
  - Sarsparilla
  - Dong Quai*
  - Black Cohosh
  - Blue Vervain
  - Red Raspberry Leaf
  - Spearmint
  - Squaw Vine
- Herbs may also relieve depression and other menopausal symptoms, such as insomnia.

Step 5a: Use supplements

- A number of vitamins and minerals are suggested to be beneficial in menopause, and there is an ever-growing market in supplements for menopausal women. There is some debate over what dosage is best and, again, this is beyond the point on the "six steps" where you can create problems as well as improvements (for example, vitamin E should be avoided in some people, including people with diabetes, heart problems or high blood pressure). ✱
  - Vitamin A is an antioxidant; it protects against cancer, builds up the immune system and is needed for healthy skin.
  - Vitamin B complex is suggested to help with hormone balancing and bone regeneration. Vitamin B6 is an anti-depressant and a diuretic.
  - Vitamin C protects against excessive bleeding and possibly cervical cancer. It is important for skin health/wound healing and helps make collagen, which is involved in bone regeneration.

- Vitamin E, another antioxidant, is thought to prevent hot flashes and protect against some kinds of cancer. It appears to be linked to the production of reproductive hormones.
- Biotin can improve the health of skin and hair; it also helps the body use EFAs.
- Magnesium is involved in bone regeneration and helps the body use enzymes.
- Zinc plays a part in hormone regulation and bone regeneration, as well as providing energy in the body.

Step 5b: Use drugs

Some of the main categories in this area include:

- Hormone replacement therapy
  - There are many brands of hormone replacement therapy (HRT) and different ways to administer this (e.g. tablets, patches or implants) but only two main types ~ combined HRT which contains oestrogen and progesterone and is the most commonly-prescribed form, and oestrogen-only HRT, which is mainly given to women who have had a hysterectomy.
  - HRT literally replaces the hormones that are decreasing in a woman's body, and thus prevents ~ or delays the onset of ~ some of the problems that some menopausal women experience.
  - Common side effects include symptoms which are similar to pre-menstrual syndrome (PMS), feeling or being sick, fluid retention, stomach cramps, putting on weight, breast tenderness, PMS type symptoms, changes in liver function (which can lead to jaundice), skin changes, altered sex drive, depression, headaches, migraines and dizziness.
  - More serious side effects include blood clots (which can lead to pulmonary embolism) and an increased chance of breast and some kinds of uterine cancer (the latter is reduced but not eliminated by combined forms of HRT). The increased risk of cancer may lead to the suggestion of additional screening tests such as mammograms, which in themselves carry risks.
- Anti-depressants
  - Work by increasing the levels of the brain chemicals called neuro-transmitters, which include noradrenaline and serotonin. Two main

kinds are used (although there are others) ~ tricyclic antidepressants and SSRI's.
- Side effects of tricyclic antidepressants include tiredness, blurred vision, drying of the mouth, constipation or difficulty in passing urine. Taking more than the prescribed amount can cause abnormal heart rhythms.
- SSRIs can cause nausea, vomiting, indigestion, diarrhoea and constipation. They can also, less commonly, cause anxiety, headache, insomnia, shaking, dizziness, dry mouth and sexual problems.
- Withdrawal symptoms can occur if anti-depressants are stopped suddenly. Symptoms include nausea, vomiting, loss of appetite, headache, dizziness, chills, insomnia, anxiety and panic.

Step 6: Break and enter

- The surgical techniques which are sometimes offered to women with menopausal problems include hysteroscopy, laparoscopy, dilation and curettage, endometrial ablation and hysterectomy, all of which are discussed in Chapter 10.
- A number of screening tests are also offered to women of menopausal age. These include cervical screening and mammograms, which are discussed further in the next chapter.

Having reached the 'serious' end of this list, which inevitably includes some of the very technical treatments available, I'd like to spiral back to the beginning of this chapter and finish with a reminder that, sometimes, the best healing comes with a nap, bubble bath, glass of wine, chat on the phone with a friend or a cuddle with a partner, child, friend, dog or cat...

Chapter 24

Beyond the Menopause

If menopause brings wisdom, which is a new or enhanced kind of knowing, then why does our society continue to use the term "old wives' tales" in such a derogatory way? As I've now said many times, our society seems to believe that medical knowledge is better than personal experience and it seems a good point to begin to explore that a bit further, by looking more closely at two ends of the spectrum ~ the aforementioned old wives' tales and the kind of 'scientific' medical knowledge which has led to the implementation of screening programmes for women, especially those who have moved beyond menopause.

The question of what actually constitutes scientific knowledge, or how we could define this, keeps hundreds of people in jobs where they research, debate and teach issues around the philosophy of science. Millions of people work as or would consider themselves scientists. So this is an incredibly multifaceted and knotty question which does not have a simple answer. Yet, given that we need a fairly simple definition to work with here, I will use what Alan Chalmers calls a 'commonsense view' of what constitutes scientific knowledge. He suggests that it is seen as knowledge "derived from the facts ... [where] the facts are presumed to be claims about the world that can be directly established by a careful, unprejudiced use of the senses" (Chalmers 1999: 1). We might add to this some of the key features of what has come to be known as the scientific 'method'; that we begin with a question or hypothesis, then collect and analyse data to see if our hypothesis is true, all the while trying to remain open to the possibility that our results might not be what we expect to see (or perhaps what we want to see).

So let's start by looking at some of those screening tests. They are commonly offered to women, sometimes once we reach a certain age, and sometimes throughout our lives. The ones that we are probably most familiar with are cervical smear testing, which attempts to detect the early stages of cervical cancer, breast examination and mammography, which both aim to detect breast cancer. As before, some of the most important questions to ask are about whether these tests are effective; whether they actually reduce the death rate from cancer. There are other questions which are equally important, like how women feel about these tests, and how many people go through the trauma of a 'false positive' result and subsequent treatment without ever having been ill, but I want to put those aside for the moment while we concentrate on the "hard" data.

Most people assumed that mammography was a useful thing to do for many years, until a few people took a hard look at the scientific data around this. Two of these people were Olsen and Gøtzsche (2004), whose work led them to draw different conclusions from those which had previously been drawn by many of their medical colleagues. They looked at seven clinical trials of mammography, which compared the causes of death in women who had screening with women who did not have screening. They concluded by saying that, "there is no reliable evidence that screening for breast cancer reduces mortality". They made a few other interesting observations about the data that they looked at:

- Not one trial of "good quality" had been carried out in this area; all of the research has been low to medium quality in relation to what is considered 'good science'. So, while they conclude that it is unjustified to continue to offer mammography screening programmes on the basis of the evidence from these trials, we might also ask why a good quality trial has not yet been conducted.
- It is misleading to use 'cause of death' as an outcome measure (the criteria by which you decide whether a treatment is useful or not), because this is a subjective decision. In other words, it is often a matter of professional medical judgement (rather than bare fact) as to exactly what caused a person's death. Furthermore, in these studies, when a woman had died from an uncertain cause, but had not had screening for breast cancer, her death was more likely to be attributed to breast cancer than if she had regular mammograms.
- It is generally accepted that, where you screen a whole population of women for breast cancer, and treat those who appear to have signs of

this, you will be treating some women who do not have a problem. Those women will face additional (unnecessary) risks by being exposed to radiation and some of them may die earlier as a result of this, for example from cardiovascular problems. However, the studies did not take this into account when they counted the numbers of 'deaths related to screening', thus making inaccurate comparisons between the risks of screening and not screening.

- Mammography screening leads to more aggressive treatment, increasing the number of mastectomies (breast removal) by about twenty per cent and the number of mastectomies and tumourectomies (tumour removal) by about thirty per cent. There are a couple of reasons for this.
  - Screening identifies some tumours that grow very slowly, and would not have caused a problem in the woman's lifetime.
  - Mammography will also detect some tumours that are not cancerous, or would not develop into invasive cancer.
- Gøtzsche also recently collaborated on a study with Jørgensen which looked at the content of web sites about mammography. They concluded that "The information material provided by professional advocacy groups and governmental organisations is information poor and severely biased in favour of screening" (Jørgensen and Gøtzsche 2004: 148).

Interestingly, although the medical journal *The Lancet* was happy to publish the review discussed above, the editor of *The Lancet* notes that the Cochrane Breast Care Cancer Group ~ the organisation who initially commissioned the work ~ disowned it (Horton 2001). He added that, "a storm of debate and criticism in national media and medical journals alike" followed the publication of the review (2001: 1294). He agrees with Olsen and Gøtzsche that, "at present, there is no reliable evidence from large randomised trials to support screening mammography programmes" (2001: 1295) and yet clearly has deep respect for the Cochrane Collaboration. He reconciles these two things by noting that, "even in the best organisations raw evidence alone is sometimes insufficient to influence opinion" (2001: 1294), reiterating the point that, as humans, often our science cannot be objective, and we find it hard to give up beliefs that we hold dear, such as the idea that screening is a beneficial thing.

In *The Whole Woman*, Greer (1999) looks at cervical screening (pap smear tests) and raises similar questions about their benefit. She listed research showing that cervical cancer had been declining well before mass screening programmes began and that the test itself has a high failure rate, which often leads to unnecessary treatment of unproven value. She goes further, in suggesting that screening tests are a way for the medical profession to exert control over women, and that they cause women to lose faith in their bodies, handing it instead to doctors.

Inevitably, she and others taking the same stance have been widely criticised. Whatever decisions we make as individual women, many people do want to hang on to the idea that screening is beneficial, in the same way that many people are attached to the idea that old wives' tales can be detrimental. I have a small collection of newspaper and magazine headlines and articles discussing old wives' tales that I've been gathering over the past few months, and the ones which appear most often illustrate the general opinion of our society:

"Fact, fiction and old wives' tales!"
"Scientists investigate old wives' tales."
"Differentiating the old wives' tales from the truth."
"Much is based on old wives' tales and misinformation..."
"This is a subject which is prone to many old wives' tales."
"Let me put a couple of old wives' tales to rest."

But then sometimes you read things which say something like,

"Like many old wives tales, this one is true."

The idea that (well-conducted) scientific studies are 'proving' the truth of some old wives' tales doesn't surprise me. I suspect that many old wives' tales were not simply yarns spun around a fire, but were snippets of knowledge drawn from trial-and-error experience and passed on down the generations. Inevitably, some may have been misinterpreted or mis-heard over the years, and some may not hold any truth at all, but I am often surprised at how quickly they are dismissed, while, as we have seen, the kind of knowledge that we see as more reliable often turns out to be peppered with problems.

It seems that, in many areas, our mums may have been right. Various scientists have shown that cranberry juice prevents the spread of bacteria that cause bladder infections and that carrots may help prevent blindness (although not necessarily night blindness, which may be one example of a tale that got altered over the years.) We have studies linking fish consumption with increased brain function, chicken soup with faster recovery from congestion, and garlic intake with lower susceptibility to colds and flu. On the other hand, research has failed to prove that chocolate gives you spots, and I can't find any studies which show a correlation between children holding sticks and an increased incidence of people getting their eyes poked out.

Not everybody is ignoring old wives' tales; a poll on babycentre.com showed that around half of the women who voted were using old wives tales to help them get pregnant, and I have been midwife to several women who enjoyed trying out the old wives' tales which are supposed to help determine the sex of your baby*. So, again, I find it difficult to understand why our mass media holds this general view that old wives' tales are poppycock, and medical knowledge holds more truth; why people shout about the old wives' tales that have now been 'disproved', or at least haven't been scientifically proven, but are less noisy about the scientific and medical beliefs which were once believed (or, perhaps, are still believed by some) and are now known to be unsubstantiated.

Chalmers' definition of science at the beginning of this chapter suggested that the broad characteristics of this were "claims about the world that can be directly established by a careful, unprejudiced use of the senses" (1999: 1). From the examples above, it could be argued that some of the old wives' tales that have been derived from years of experience, trial and error are more authentically scientific than the information women are given about mammograms. I don't suppose any 'old wife' ever had anything much to gain from the idea that chicken soup prevented colds; she would probably have been happy to switch her allegiance to vegetable soup, or beef stew, if these had proven more successful over the years.

---

* The two basic suggestions are for the woman to eat foods high in sodium and potassium for a girl, and calcium and magnesium for a boy, and to make love two or three days before ovulation for a girl, and between one day before and a few hours after ovulation for a boy.

These 'old wives' did, however, have much to gain from learning from their experience and using 'trial and error' to try to determine the answers to questions that would help increase the length of their own lives and those of their children.

Medical screening programmes are primarily about populations; the only way they can cater to the individual is when they are run by kind, caring people who have the time, energy and compassion to talk through the issues with every single woman who walks through the door of the clinic. Women's stories, on the other hand, are primarily personal, although sometimes those stories become collective enough to be passed on through the years. Whether or not you place your faith in science, Western medicine, women's wisdom or all of the above, there is one thing that cannot be denied. The cost of the breast screening programme in the UK in 1999/2000 (which are the latest figures available, so the real cost is likely to have increased) was £52 million. That is not a misprint, fifty-two million pounds was spent on screening tests which some experts have shown are a waste of time and money. Whether you agree with them or not, there is no arguing with the fact that this would be more than enough to pay for a few luxury menopause hotels where older women could sit around and come up with more individual and collective wisdom for some of those millions of scientists to check.

Chapter 25

Returning to the Wheel

"The wise King Yudhishthir was once asked what the greatest wonder in the world was. He famously replied that the greatest wonder was that every day men see creatures go to the realm of Yama (the Lord of Death) and yet those who remain seek to live forever (Buck 1981). Singh (1998) echoes this point, observing that while acknowledging that death awaits them, many people actually behave as though an exception will be made in their case. Death can cause panic and is something our modern culture would rather not think about until forced to (Mitterrand 1997)."

(Sheran 2004, unpublished essay)

I borrowed the paragraph above from my partner, who recently did some work on death and spirituality. I had sat at my computer for a full fifteen minutes, unable to think of an opening line for this chapter. Perhaps it is too late in the day, perhaps it is time for me to take my own advice and have a rest from the work spiral, or perhaps it is that I, too, am feeling the effects of being the product of a culture which finds it immensely difficult to bring up the subject of death. Yet death, like birth, is one of the few transition points on the spiral of life that we will all experience, and it surely therefore deserves our attention just as much as the other transitions of our being.

In our modern medically focused culture, death is often seen as a failure rather than a part of life. In English, we have lots of metaphors which prevent us from having to say the words "death", "dying" or "dead" if we want to avoid them. Where I use the word birth freely throughout this book, for some reason I chose a metaphor for the title of this chapter rather than calling it something like "Dying and Death". Perhaps it is because, in our society, dying and suffering are generally considered 'bad', while being alive and healthy are considered 'good'. Yet, unless any of us can find a way to join that small group of spiritual leaders like Rama, Krishna, Jesus and Elijah, who were said to ascend with their physical bodies, death is a reality of life.

It is a reality within which we can choose to be comfortable, electing to live our lives every day to the full, or with which we can choose to be uncomfortable and fear-filled. Much of what we call 'preventative medicine', which is so popular with our contemporary healers, aims to prolong life and inhibit death, and it is certainly possible to tap into a lot of death-related fear in our modern world. Yet if we spend our whole lives doing things which are aimed at preventing our deaths, we may reach death and realise that we haven't really enjoyed living. As Bernie Siegel said in an interview with Peyser (1998):

> *"I tell people, don't do things to not die, it doesn't work. If you meditate, eat vegetables, and jog, so that you won't die, you'll be very upset some day that you didn't sleep late, and have a steak, and an ice cream cone. I do things because I feel good living a certain way. So I exercise and I meditate, and I love ~ because I like living that way. Now I know that it makes me younger than somebody else my age. But I'm not doing it to put off dying. I'm doing it because I really enjoy living. I look forward to dying, as an experience, someday."*

There is really no knowing exactly how we will die ahead of time; although there is plenty of data out there which shows what percentage of the population are likely to die of what cause. It is not hard to find quizzes which allow you to put in a few bits of information about your lifestyle (diet, smoking habits, exercise levels and family health history) which will allow you to calculate how long you can expect to live, barring accidents. Perhaps inevitably, I can't find a study which looks at whether these are accurate!

Yet mortality data is based on what doctors write on death certificates, and, as in the previous chapter, causes of death are not always certain ~ they are subjective opinions. Some conditions are not easily recognised, or may not be known about, and others may carry social stigma and therefore be less likely to be recorded. Clarke and Gladwin (2001) found that the doctors they interviewed saw the filling out of death certificates as a "necessary evil" which interrupted them from their "real work". They urge doctors to take more care in their recording of cause of death, alongside the suggestion that medical students should be encouraged to think about what a "good death" might be, in order to improve care for those who are still living.

There are some interesting parallels between the places where people are born and the places where people die. For almost all of human history, until only a few decades ago, most people were born at home and died at home. This has now almost completely turned around, so that the most common place to be born or to die is in hospital. In fact, it could be said that the hospital is now the accepted place for both birth and death, which is one reason why even those women who feel rationally that they are safer giving birth in the hospital actually feel unsafe on a deeper, more primal level; I have looked after several women having their babies in hospital who had only ever been to a hospital before when someone they loved was dying.

A very few people will always accidentally be born in random places, like the back of taxis or in supermarkets, perhaps because their mothers had no sensations which let them know they were in labour or because they came earlier than they were expected. Equally, a larger proportion of people will also die accidentally in random places ~ again, often because they took this journey earlier than they might have expected. In both cases, whether or not birth or death is inevitable, and even if the person has already been born or has died, they will usually be rushed to hospital. In our society, this is taken as read; paramedics are obliged to take people to the hospital, even if they might prefer, given a choice, to be taken home. While many people may be happy going to the hospital, wanting to know that everything possible was done in order to try and prevent death, and mechanisms are in place which mean that hospital workers are generally respectful of the wishes of the person and her family around withholding treatment, it is curious that we don't, as a society, offer people a choice of where they would like to die if their death comes suddenly.

There are alternative places to die if death comes at the end of a terminal illness; those working in the hospice movement have created incredibly peaceful, loving environments for people to spend their last days, perhaps because they need more care than can be given at home. It has always surprised me that the birth centre movement, which aims to do the same thing in providing a home-like environment for birthing women and their families, has not received as much attention, funding and support from politicians and the general public as the hospice movement.

Perhaps we should consider giving the decision around where we would like to die as much attention as the decision around where we would like to give birth, or be born. In Chapter 5, I raised some questions about how you would like to be greeted if you were travelling to a new world in a spaceship. Here, the questions are more about how you would like to prepare for your journey. Of course, some of us won't get to make those choices, but, if you could choose, would you like to get ready in your own home with your family, friends and familiar things around, or would you like to be in an institution with others who were going on a similar journey? Would you like to be "out of it", oblivious to the transition, or would you like to be as fully conscious and aware for as long as you could be?

For some people, terminal illness brings about incredible spiritual growth. In his last interview, Dennis Potter spoke of his feeling of serenity and of the "nowness" of everything. His ability to focus on the present moment, rather than looking back into the past or forward into the future, only came through when he knew he was approaching death. Many people have been shocked and appalled to hear a doctor give them a terminal diagnosis, only to find that this was the trigger they needed to release fear or other things that they felt had been holding them back:

> "There were those ... whose dying expressed a wholeness of being; their hearts were so open, their spirits so fully released that it was evident how well they had become during the weeks and months of their dying... They were more healed, more whole at the moment of their dying than at any time in their life. They had healed into death, their business finished, their future wide open."
>
> (Levine 1989: 5)

Search any mind, body and spirit shelf in a bookstore and you will find several accounts of how people used deadly illness to bring them "back to life" and learn or develop healing techniques which have been successful enough to sell thousands of books and bring hope to others in similar situations. This is not to say, however, that we will all choose to die gracefully, or with increased spiritual insights; two of the women I talked to mentioned that their loved ones became more angry and difficult to be with as they died, and there is a need to honour that this may be the kind of journey that some people choose. Some people, when facing death, find that being urged to open themselves to transcendence and see the positive good that stems from suffering simply feel annoyed: it is easy for those of us who can see no end to our lives to urge others to change.

While we can choose how we face our own journey, our own thoughts on what a good birth or death may be like might not work for other people.

We all believe different things about what happens to us after we die. Over time, the different death and burial rites of cultures have aligned with a variety of beliefs. Ancient Egyptians chose mummification, Neolithic Pagans chose to be painted in red ochre and buried in a fetal position; modern Christians may choose to be buried in a churchyard or under a cross. We no longer live in tribes where everybody's beliefs are similar, and somehow we have ended up in a situation where death and birth are relatively standardised events which are dealt with by professionals who may not be known to us.

Around both death and birth, medical professionals are often happy to embrace spiritual beliefs as long as they don't interfere with clinical outcomes, but, as Rumbold (2000) suggests, they may balk at beliefs and wishes which lead to non-compliance with their suggested treatments. Perhaps some people find it hard to understand why people who face a terminal diagnosis would choose to refuse further treatment in order that they can go home and die among their own family. It might be equally difficult for some to understand why the parents of a baby who has a condition which means they won't live more than a few hours following birth might choose to give birth at home. Yet, for some people, making these choices ensure that these transitions are more sacred and special for those who are living and dying through them.

Drawing parallels between birth and death is certainly not a new idea. Midwives used to take care of dying people and lay out the dead. In many ways, it is a shame that this does not happen now; the ability of a good midwife to be with someone on their journey, understanding that this is the person's journey and not the midwife's is just as applicable when this journey is towards birth or death. If birth can be a sacred rite of passage, then why not death? We might not feel that we are able to consciously control how we die ~ although some people certainly believe that we create our own choices on some level ~ but we can choose to face the reality that we will die and think about how we would like this to be for us, while embracing the joy of life, chocolate, too much wine and all of the other things that help us enjoy ourselves while we are here.

Chapter 26

The Cycle Continues

Whether we're looking at birth, death, or any of the spirals which women experience in between, there is so much more to explore than many people are aware of. By looking at how Western society's attitudes towards women's cycles and spirals have changed throughout time, we can step aside from the definitions, attitudes and assumptions held by our modern culture and take a wider view on whether these are empowering or constraining. By taking a look at what it is to be in the centre of an experience, such as being born, or mothering a child, we can reframe the choices we have to make in relation to the lived experiences of those journeys, rather than simply following the 'average' path, which may not be the one which suits us as an individual.

By thinking about how we 'know' things, we can see that science, while being a useful tool for generating information around some aspects of our experiences, is just one of many ways of knowing, and that we truly are the experts of our own individual bodies. Ultimately, by putting all of these things together, we can see that, while it is a fantastic thing that we, as a society, have the ability to 'break and enter' when this is truly the only option, there are many other things we can do for ourselves (or that other types of healers can do with us) when we experience problems.

There are some general themes which arise from this exploration, including the suggestion that women experience different aspects of their brains during different times of their menstrual cycle, and perhaps during different times of their life in general. I don't know whether all woman have the potential to experience a different kind of reality during menstruation, pregnancy and menopause, or whether this idea has developed as a way of simply allowing women more space at this time. However, as I have said before, continuing to extol rationality as better than any other way of being and knowing is not going to take us nearly as far as if we could stay open to other possibilities. Perhaps we need to stop seeing the opposite of rational as being "irrational", which is perceived negatively in our culture, and see it as being intuitive, insightful or creative around knowledge.

In *The Seat of the Soul*, Gary Zukav (1990) talked about the difference between five-sensory human beings and multi-sensory human beings. The distinction, he says, is in whether we believe solely that truth and experience come through our five senses from the physical world, or whether we believe that there are other dimensions of our existence, such as the soul, which we experience in ways other than through our five senses. We appear to be living in a time when, while there are some people who would dismiss this outright, multi-sensory ways of knowing are, for other people, becoming a powerful force which helps them to grow and make choices.

Some of the themes which arose when I was talking to women and reading what others had written included the idea that women need to make spaces for themselves ∼ sometimes literally, sometimes figuratively ∼ and the power of transitions, or in-between times. When we look at a spiral drawn on paper, we tend to focus on the line, on the spiral itself, yet there is another spiral made by the space between the lines. Only by honouring women's spaces, including our own, will we get to explore what the in-between might be about. No wonder, then, that some women are finding value in drumming while they bleed, planting gardens while they bloom in pregnancy, birthing in spaces they create themselves, reframing their lives as they reach what we call 'middle-age' and actively attempting to switch off their rational brain while they paint their menopausal journey.

They are also choosing different ways of teaching their daughters about the sacredness of their own cycles:

> "My mother never explained to me why I had them. She just said, 'this happens to you, it's not very nice'. I felt dirty and I think it made me feel that it was something you didn't talk about openly and certainly not with men. I've brought up my kids differently and they are both fine with that. They know all about it."

> (Phoebe)

"I wouldn't have done it in the same way. I felt dismissed when I asked my own mum. I obviously wouldn't do that to my own children. You know, if and when I have daughters, I would sit down and tell them it's a wonderful thing. And, yes, you might have some pains at certain times but it's actually a wonderful thing."

(Olivia)

"I would just try and put it into perspective. I think it's the secrecy thing that did my head in."

(Mieke)

"I want to buy a special gift for my daughter when she first bleeds. Maybe even one of those stone goddesses that you put a drop of your first blood in. And maybe take her out to dinner. And, if I thought she'd like it, I'd have a women's circle and ask everybody to share their experiences with her."

(Freya)

Just one example of how we are learning new things about women every day is provided by some recent work that was carried out in California. It is well understood within certain disciplines which use scientific methods (though not always outside of them) that women and female animals have often been overlooked in research, sometimes because it is deemed easier to use male animals or humans in research because they do not have menstrual cycles and hormonal fluctuations which apparently make research more difficult (Goodman 1994).

This was certainly the case for the research looking at how people became stressed, and how they coped with stress, about ninety per cent of which has been carried out on men. This would be fine if we knew for sure that men and women behaved in similar ways but, as some of the studies discussed in other chapters have shown, this is not always the case. Historically, studies on stress have led to the development of a theory that people tend to have a "fight or flight" reaction, when they encounter stressful situations; their bodies get ready for them to either fight something, or run away. Supposedly, this stems from times when we might occasionally face hungry animals and needed to develop ways of activating our bodies to move quickly.

This 'fight or flight' response is not necessarily missing in women; women have been known to lift heavy cars off a trapped child, reach Olympic running speeds when needing to rescue a child in trouble in water, and, as any midwife will tell you, to stop their labour through the release of adrenaline if they feel unsafe in their environment. Yet Klein and Taylor followed a hunch with research that showed that women may have a whole repertoire of responses to stress, which includes one they call "tend and befriend" (Taylor et al 2000).

The two women noticed that when the women scientists they worked with were stressed, they did not go off and seek solitude ('flight') like their male colleagues; instead, they came into the lab, cleaned, made coffee, and spent time 'bonding' with other women. Sure enough, when they researched this apparent difference, they discovered that women respond to stress by releasing chemicals that are more likely to encourage us to 'make friends' and spend time with other women than run away and hide by ourselves. This befriending, in turn, means we release more oxytocin (which is perhaps linked to the synchronisation of women's menstrual cycles, although that was not part of their study) and reduces our stress further. Men, on the other hand, produce testosterone when they are stressed, which seems to reduce the effects of oxytocin.

These researchers even suggest that it is because women 'tend and befriend' that we consistently live longer than men. Our women friends, it seems, help us to live longer, better, happier lives. Yet most women won't need to be told this; it is something we intuitively know. Many women learn as teenagers that their friends will be with them after their current relationship has broken up, and women of all ages who encounter friends with problems tend to respond by making tea, offering sympathy and, sometimes, by gathering other women around to offer support. How amazing that, even though Western attitudes have sometimes encouraged individual women to be competitive and at odds with each other, when a crisis occurs, we tend to forget our differences, gather together, and 'befriend'.

Chapter 27

Reclaiming the Spiral

Dans quelle langue respirait ta grand-mère?

Même après plusieurs siècles
et des milliers de refuges,
elle vente toujours sa patte
sur les parois de nos gorges,
rugueuses,
nord-américaines.
Ramassée et ressassée
de jupons en tabliers,
haletée par nos ancêtres
alors qu'elles nous portaient
de soupir en inhalation,
de génération en génération
dans l'abîme de leurs corps

In what language did your grandmother breathe?

Even after many centuries
and a thousand retreats
she still winds her paw
on the hills of our throats
rugged
north american
picked up and swished around
from petticoats to aprons
panted by our elders
as they carried us
from sighs to inhalations
from generation to generation
in the abyss of their bodies

Sophie Bérubé (2002)

My mum is one of those women who, when you ask what she would like for her birthday, will tell you she already has everything she needs. So, when her sixtieth birthday approached, I decided that, instead of buying her a present, I would make her something that she could keep. I decided to ask some of the women in her life if they would send me a small piece of fabric, and then make her a patchwork quilt (which I imagined would hang on the wall) out of whatever I received. Not knowing what kind of response I would get, I set about tentatively making some phone calls to some of the women in our family, and a few of her close friends.

The entire process (which, as I begin to write this chapter, is still ongoing) seemed such an amazing illustration of how incredible women are that it seemed natural for this story of a patchwork quilt to become the final chapter of a patchwork book. Within an hour of making the first few phone calls, to see what people thought about the idea, I had a small group of women who were already planning what they would send me, and who had offered to phone some others. That evening, I made a list to keep a record of the women that I had spoken to and the women that had offered to call for me. My sister had helped me compile a list of some of the women we knew, and had her own list of people to call. My dad also knew about the project and was waiting for an opportunity to call me when my mum went out, as I imagined that he would be able to give me many of the phone numbers I needed.

By the next day, the list was so long that it had to be transferred to a much larger piece of paper. There were already about thirty women's names on the list, although I didn't expect that they would all send fabric, given how busy women are these days. The list itself had turned into a web, as each woman promised to pass the message on to others, some of whom passed it on again. Each time I spoke to any of the women who was involved, they would tell me whom else they had talked to, and more names would be added. At the centre of the web was a spiral, with arms going off into different areas of my mother's life; an arm of sisters and relatives; an arm of friends from her working days; an arm of friends from sports clubs. Soon, the spirals began to weave themselves together, as friends from one area of her life bumped into friends from another and told each other about the project, only to find out they both already knew!

Two days after I began making my calls, my dad still hadn't had a chance to call me, yet the web had over sixty names on it. At that point, I had only spoken to fifteen women, and eight of those were women who lived in other countries, or whom I knew wouldn't be able to call anyone else. It was a core of seven women who had managed to spread the word, almost overnight, to more than sixty others. You don't have to look for in our culture to find derogatory references made about women spending too much time on the telephone; yet this, if nothing else, demonstrates just how effective a small group of women with a telephone each can be! During this project, I thought a lot about how effective women are in passing news, information and knowledge on to each other; women's "word of mouth" is probably a far better way to advertise than television! Women are a powerful force, in communication, and in action.

On the second day I also started to receive fabric through the post, and, for the next three weeks, there wasn't one day when I didn't receive fabric from at least two women. On the days when my partner got up before me, he would bring the mail upstairs, and I would excitedly open envelopes and spread the fabric out on the bed. I had always known that my mum had lots of friends, but it was amazing to discover just how many women were willing to respond so quickly, to find fabric, put it in the post, and essentially send a piece of themselves to another woman. I had originally thought about drawing a map of the quilt itself, and writing the women's names in the squares that they had sent, so my mum would know who sent what. But the whole thing felt so much like I was being sent love for my mum, that I started cutting a small heart out of each piece of fabric and putting it in a photo album with the name of the woman it had come from beside it.

By the time my dad was able to call me (when my mum finally went out for a few minutes!), almost all of the women whose numbers I thought I would need had already been contacted. There were already almost ninety names, and the numbers he provided took the total to over a hundred. In total, I received one hundred and four pieces of fabric, including offerings from four lady cats! The project became inter-generational, with fabric arriving from mothers and daughters, baby girls, children, teenagers, young women, older women, mothers, grandmothers and great-grandmothers.

Some women sent pieces of fabric that had been bought specially; one said she stood in the aisle at the craft shop, brought my mother to mind and waited to see what jumped out at her. Others sent pieces of fabric they already had that were meaningful to them. Curtains became a recurring theme; I received two or three remnants from the curtains in rooms where my mum has spent happy evenings, and fabric which had been miraculously found in the attic from some curtains that my mum made for another friend over thirty years before. I received fabric from a much loved blouse, which no longer fitted but brought happy memories; the spare fabric from the blanket made for the puppy that came along to celebrate a new love; and the hat that my grandmother wore for my mum and dad's wedding some thirty-eight years ago.

Often, as I looked at the map, this web of the women in my mother's life, I thought about all of the other webs that connected with it. Each of the women in my mum's web has a whole web of their own as well, as does each of the women whose words are in this book, and each of the webs has shared connections, making every woman ~ and man ~ in the world a part of the same web. I always liked the film, "How to Make a American Quilt", whose tagline can be found at the beginning of Chapter 1. The film itself is about a group of women who share their stories with a younger woman who is at a crossroads in her life. If each of the pieces in the patchwork could tell the stories of the woman who sent it, then it would be a rich source of knowledge indeed.

Coincidentally (or perhaps not, if you think about it in a multi-sensory way), I was finishing this book at the same time I was finishing my mum's quilt. I learned new ways to take my own advice about spiralling in the ways that work for us as individuals. When my body let me know I had been sitting at the computer too long, or when I was stuck for what to write next, I would move downstairs or into the garden and sew some more patches into the quilt. And sometimes, as I sewed, the answer to the question I had been pondering would come to me, and I would finish the patch I was working on, and come back upstairs to write.

It was a curious thing too, to be writing this book while also talking to some of the women in my mum's life, as well as the women I've been interviewing, whose stories are in here. I knew before I started that I could only really hope to scratch the surface in this book; that the real stories, and the real sacredness of women's spirals are out there in women's lives, not on paper. I knew that, as women have always told their stories orally, it was something of a misnomer to try to *write* about women's spirals. Because our spirals cannot really be captured on paper; they are in our lives, our cycles, our bodies, our experiences. Maybe one day, when we have moved further on in our ways of knowing, we will have better ways of expressing these things to ourselves and each other.

Women are amazing creatures. We bear incredible hardships ourselves, and bring incredible joy to others. We can heal ourselves when we are sick, and nurture each other when we're together. We have arms that can make our lovers feel as safe as when they were with their own mother, laps that can hold several children at once, breasts that can feed babies and kisses that can cure anything. We are made of the softest substance of the universe when we need to give love or cuddles, and the hardest substance in the universe when we need to stand up to something or somebody who is hurting someone we love. We have vital truths, and incredible knowledge, which we willingly share with others.

There is really only one thing that is wrong with women, and it is that we often forget our own worth. We forget how valuable we are, to others and ourselves, we forget how well our bodies carry out their responsibilities (even if they are sometimes only being nourished by bits and pieces which we found at the back of the fridge because we are too busy feeding others to feed ourselves properly), and we forget how much the world depends on us. If we could only remember how very valuable, powerful and essential we are to the running of the planet, and how well our bodies work to enable us to do all of these things, I suspect that everything else would probably follow.

References

Abercrombie N (1988). *Dictionary of Sociology*. London: Penguin.

Angier N (1999). *Woman: An Intimate Geography*. Boston: Houghton Mifflin.

Arms S (1994). *Immaculate Deception II*. Berkeley, CA: Celestial Arts.

Baskett T and Nagele F (2000). Naegele's rule: a reappraisal. *British Journal of Obstetrics and Gynaecology*, 107: 1433–1435.

Beech BAL and Robinson J (1994). *Ultrasound? Unsound*. London: AIMS; available from www.aims.org.uk/aims.htm

Belenky MF, Clinchy BMV, Goldberger NR and Tarule JM (1997). *Women's Ways of Knowing: The Development of Self, Voice and Mind*. New York, NY: Basic Books.

Bennett P (1993). Critical clitoridectomy: female sexual imagery and feminist psychoanalytic theory. *Signs: Journal of Women in Culture and Society*, 18: 235–259.

Bergsjo P, Daniel W, Denman III DW et al. (1990). Duration of human singleton pregnancy; a population-based study. *Acta Obstetrica Gynecologica Scandinavica*, 69: 197–207.

Bérubé S (2002). *La Trombe Sacrée*. More information on the book can be found at http://www3.sympatico.ca/ed.david/li-trombe-sacree.html or http://livres.info.ca/livres2.cfm?cat=livres&souscategorieid=8 (French).

Brook D (1976). *Nature-Birth*. London: Penguin.

Brooks-Gunn J and Matthews WS (1979). *He and She: How Children Develop Their Sex Role Identity*. Englewood, NJ: Prentice-Hall.

Buck W (1981). *Mahabharata*. California: University of California Press.

Case AM and Reid RL (1998). Effects of the menstrual cycle on medical disorders. *Archives of Internal Medicine*, 158: 1405–1412.

Chalmers I, Enkin M and Kierse MJNC (Eds) (1989). *Effective Care in Pregnancy and Childbirth*. Oxford: Oxford University Press.

Chamberlain D (2003). *Life Before Birth: Introduction*. http://www.birthpsychology.com/lifebefore/index.html

Clarke A and Gladwin J (2003). In search of a good death. *British Medical Journal* 327: 221.

Coad J and Dunstall M (2001). *Anatomy and Physiology for Midwives*. Edinburgh: Mosby.

Coney S (1995). *The Menopause Industry: A Guide to Medicine's Discovery of the Mid-life Woman*. London: The Women's Press.

Cooper LS, Gillett CE, Patel NK, Barnes DM and Fentimen IS (1999). Survival of premenopausal breast carcinoma patients in relation to menstrual cycle timing of surgery and estrogen-receptor/progesterone-receptor status of the primary tumor. *Cancer*, 86(10): 2053–2058.

Davis E (2000). *Women's Sexual Passages*. Berkeley, CA: Hunter House.

Davis E and Leonard C (1997). *The Women's Wheel of Life. Thirteen Archetypes of Woman at Her Fullest Power*. New York: Penguin Arkana.

Davis-Floyd RE (1992). *Birth As an American Rite of Passage*. Berkeley: University of California Press.

Deutsch B (2004). *The Male Privilege Checklist*. An Unabashed Imitation of an Article by Peggy McIntosh. http://www.expositorymagazine.net/maleprivilege_checklist.php

Diamant A (2002). *The Red Tent*. London: Pan Books.

Dick-Read G (1942). *Childbirth Without Fear*. London: Heinemann Medical.

Duerk J (1989). *Circle of Stones: Woman's Journey to Herself*. Philadelphia: Innisfree Press.

Eisler R (1988). *The Chalice and the Blade. Our History, Our Future*. San Fransisco, CA: HarperCollins.

England P and Horowitz R (1998). *Birthing From Within. An Extra-ordinary Guide to Childbirth Preparation*. Albuquerque: Partera Press.

Ensler E (2002). *The Vagina Monologues*. London: Virago.

Erdrich L (1995). *The Blue Jay's Dance: A Birth Year*. New York: HarperCollins.

Estés CP (1996). A walk in El Rio Abajo Rio. In: Bonnie JH (Ed.) *Red Moon Passage: The Power and Wisdom of Menopause*. London: Thorsons.

Flint C, Poulengeris P and Grant A (1989). The know your midwife scheme ~ a randomised trial of continuity of care by a team of midwives. *Midwifery* 5: 11–16.

Gaskin IM (1990). *Spiritual Midwifery*, 3rd edition. Summertown, TN: The Book Publishing Company.

Gaskin IM (2003). *Ina May's Guide to Childbirth*. New York: Bantam.

Giddens A (1987). *Social Theory and Modern Sociology*. Cambridge: Cambridge University Press.

Gilligan C (1993). *In a Different Voice. Psychological Theory and Women's Development*, 2nd edition. Cambridge, MA: Harvard University Press.

Goodman E (1994). Research that ignores females is no bargain. In: Hicks KM (Ed.) *Misdiagnosis: Woman as a Disease*. Allentown, PA: People's Medical Society.

Gøtzsche PC and Olsen O (2000). Is screening for breast cancer with mammography justifiable? *The Lancet*, 355: 129–134.

Grahn J (1993). *Blood, Bread and Roses. How Menstruation Created the World.* Boston, MA: Beacon Press.

Green JM (1993). Expectations and experiences of pain in labor: findings from a large prospective study. *Birth*, 20(2): 65–72.

Greer G (1999). *The Whole Woman*. London: Doubleday.

Harrison A (1991). Childbirth in Kuwait: the experiences of three groups of Arab mothers. *Journal of Pain and Symptom Management*, 6: 466–475.

Horton R (2001). Screening mammography ~ an overview revisited. *The Lancet*, 358(9290): 1284–1285.

Hylan TR, Sundell K and Judge R (1999). The impact of premenstrual symptomatology on functioning and treatment-seeking behavior: experience from the United States, United Kingdom, and France. *Journal of Women's Health and Gender-Based Medicine*, 8(8): 1043–1052.

Illich I (1990). *Limits to Medicine; Medical Nemesis, the Expropriation of Health.* London: Penguin.

Jaggar AM (1988). *Feminist Politics and Human Nature*. New Jersey: Rowman and Littlefield.

Jonas E. Eugen Jonas' web site can be found at www.centrum.jonas.com and you can find many of the sceptical responses to his work simply by putting his name into an Internet search engine.

Jørgensen KJ and Gøtzsche PC (2004). Presentation on websites of possible benefits and harms from screening for breast cancer: cross sectional study. *British Medical Journal*, 328: 148.

Kohlberg L (1969). *Stages in the Development of Moral Thought*. New York: Holt, Rinehart.

Lacy L (1974). *Lunaception*. New York: Warner Books.

Lahdenperä M, Lummaa V, Helle S, Tremblay M and Russell AF (2004). Fitness benefits of prolonged post-reproductive lifespan in women. *Nature*, 128(11): 178–181.

Leonard C (1999). Women of the thirteenth moon: the menopause experience ~ Part 1. *Birth Gazette*, 15(2): 39–47.

Levine S (1989). *Healing into Life and Death*. Bath: Gateway Books.

Luminaire-Rosen C (2000). *Parenting Begins Before Conception. A guide to Preparing Mind, Body and Spirit for You and Your Future Child*. Rochester, VT: Healing Arts Press.

McCourt C and Page L (1996). *Report on the Evaluation of One-to-One Midwifery*. London: The Hammersmith Hospital NHS Trust and Thames Valley University.

McLintock MK (1971). Menstrual synchrony and suppression. *Nature*, 229: 5282.

Mead M, cited on http://www.voiceofwomen.com/articles/menopauseart.html

Mitchell DP (1996). Postmodernism, health and illness. *Journal of Advanced Nursing*, 23: 201–205.

Mitterrand F (1997). In: De Hennezel M (Ed.) *Intimate Death*. London: Warner Books.

Mittendorf R, Williams MA, Berkey CS et al. (1990). The length of uncomplicated human gestation. *Obstetrics and Gynecology*, 75: 929–932.

Morse JM and Park C (1988). Differences in cultural expectations of the perceived painfulness of childbirth. In: Michaelson KL (Ed.) *Childbirth in America: Anthropological Perspectives*. South Hadley, MA: Bergin & Garvey; pp. 121–129.

Natale V, Albertazzi P and Cangini A (2003). The effects of menstrual cycle on dreaming. *Biological Rhythm Research*, 34(3): 295–303.

O'Connell HE, Hutson JM, Anderon CR and Plenter RJ (1998). Anatomical relationship between urethra and clitoris. *Journal of Urology*, 159(6): 1892–1897.

Odent M (2001). *The Scientification of Love*. London: Free Association Books.

Olsen O and Gøtzsche PC (2001). Cochrane review on screening for breast cancer with mammography. *The Lancet*, 358(9290): 1340–1342.

Palmer G (2004). Feminism and breastfeeding. In: Stewart M (Ed.) *Pregnancy, Birth and Maternity Care: Feminist Perspectives*. Oxford: Books for Midwives; pp. 85–104.

Pathanapong P (1990). Childbirth Pain in Communicative Behaviors among Selected Laboring Thai Women. Tempe, AZ: University of Arizona. Unpublished doctoral dissertation.

Peyser R (1998). *An Interview with Bernie Siegel*. http://members.aol.com/rpeyser/siegel.htm

Prendeville W, Harding J, Elbourne D et al. (1988). The Bristol third stage trial: active versus physiological management of the third stage of labour. *British Medical Journal*, 297: 1295–1300.

Reynolds PC (1991). *Stealing Fire: The Mythology of the Technocracy*. Palo Alto, CA: Iconic Anthropology Press.

Robbins J (1996). *Reclaiming Our Health*. California: HJ Kramer.

Rooks JP, Weatherby NL and Ernst EKM (1992). The National Birth Center Study. *Journal of Nurse-Midwifery*, 37(5): 301–330.

Rosser J (2000). Calculating the EDD; which is more accurate, scan or LMP? *The Practising Midwife*, 3(3): 28–29.

Rubin JZ, Provenzano FJ and Luria Z (1974). The eye of the beholder: parents' views on sex of newborns. *American Journal of Orthopsychiatry*, 44: 4.

Rumbold B (2002). *Spirituality and Palliative Care: Social and Pastoral Perspectives*. Oxford: Oxford University Press.

SARK (1997). *Succulent Wild Woman*. Dancing with your wonder-full self. Simon and Schuster, New York; SARK's web site can be found at www.campsark.com

Schiebinger L (1987). History and philosophy. In: Harding S and O'Barr JF (Eds) *Sex and Scientific Inquiry*. Chicago: University of Chicago Press.

Sheran I (2004). Dying to be Healed? Spiritual Transformation at the End of Life. Unpublished essay.

Singh K (1998). *The Grace in Dying: How We Are Transformed Spiritually As We Die*. Dublin: Newleaf.

Sjöö M and Mor B (1987). *The Great Cosmic Mother ~ Rediscovering the Religion of the Earth*. San Francisco: HarperCollins.

Smith C and Lloyd B (1978). Maternal behavior and perceived sex of infant: revisited. *Child Development*, 49: 1263–1265.

Spretnak C (1993). Foreword. In: Judy Grahn (Ed.) *Blood, Bread and Roses. How Menstruation Created the World*. Boston, MA: Beacon Press.

Starhawk (1990). *Dreaming the Dark: Magic, Sex and Politics*. London: Unwin.

Steingraber S (2001). *Having Faith: An Ecologist's Journey to Motherhood*. New York: Perseus Publishing.

Taylor SE, Klein LC, Lewis BP, Gruenewald TL, Gurung RAR and Updegraff JA (2000). Female responses to stress: tend and be friend, not fight or flight. *Psychological Review*, 107(3): 411–429.

Tew M (1985). Place of birth and perinatal mortality. *Journal of the Royal College of General Practitioners*, August 1995, 35: 390–394.

Vincent Priya J (1992). *Birth Traditions and Modern Pregnancy Care*. Shaftesbury: Element.

Weed SS (1989). *Healing Wise*. Woodstock, NY: Ash Tree Publishing; Susun's web site can be found at www.susunweed.com

Weisenberg M and Caspi Z (1989). Cultural and educational influences on pain of childbirth. *Journal of Pain and Symptom Management*, 4: 13–19.

Wickham S (1999). Further thoughts on the third stage. *Practising Midwife*, 2(10): 14–15. Reprinted in *MIDIRS Midwifery Digest*, 10(2): 204–205 and at www.withwoman.co.uk

Wickham S (2002). *What's Right For Me? Making Decisions in Pregnancy and Birth*. London: AIMS.

Wickham S (2004). Feminism and ways of knowing. In: Stewart M (Ed.) *Pregnancy, Birth and Maternity Care: Feminist Perspectives*. Oxford: Books for Midwives; pp. 157–168.

Zerubavel E (1985). *The Seven Day Circle*. Chicago, IL: University of Chicago Press.

Resources

This book has a sister web page with links to resources on the Internet: please click on the "Sacred Cycles" link on www.withwoman.co.uk

Menstrual choices

To find out more about alternatives...

Women's Environmental Network
P.O. Box 30626, London E1 1TZ, UK
Tel.: +44 (0)20 7481 9004
Fax: +44 (0)20 7481 9144
http://www.wen.org.uk/sanpro/sanpro.htm

There are also a few commercial web sites online where you can look at the products and see testimonials...

http://www.lunapads.com
http://www.birthwithsol.com/fehy.html

Great birth books

Some of the books offering information on birth choices which have not been already cited here include:

Beverley B (2004). *Am I allowed? Yes, Yes Yes!* London: AIMS.
Henci G and Rhonda W (1999). *The Thinking Woman's Guide to a Better Birth*. Perigee Books.
Sheila K (2000). *Rediscovering Birth*. Little, Brown & Co.

Organisations promoting choice in childbirth

Association for Improvements in the Maternity Services (AIMS)
5 Ann's Court, Grove Road, Surbiton, Surrey KT6 4BE, UK
AIMS Helpline: +44 0870 7651433
chair@aims.org.uk

Association of Radical Midwives (ARM)
62a Greetby Hill, Ormskirk, Lancashire, England L39 2DT, UK
+44 01695 572776
arm@radmid.demon.co.uk

Independent Midwives Association (IMA)
1 The Great Quarry, Guildford, England GU1 3XN, UK
+44 01483 821104
www.independentmidwives.co.uk

National Childbirth Trust (NCT)
Alexandra House, Oldham Terrace, London, England W3 6NH, UK
Enquiry Line: +44 0870 444 8707

Useful birth-related web sites

www.aims.org.uk
www.davis-floyd.com
www.inamay.com
www.independentmidwives.org.uk
www.midirs.org
www.midwiferytoday.com
www.radmid.demon.co.uk
www.rebirth.dk/hbr/birth.htm
www.sheilakitzinger.com
www.susunweed.com
www.withwoman.co.uk

More web sites to explore

www.planetsark.com
www.famouscreativewomen.com
www.menopause-metamorphosis.com
www.selfesteem4women.com
www.womansource.com
www.fwhc.org
www.moonsurfing.com

Happy exploring!

Index of Names

Subject Index